LONG TERM CARE NURSES GUIDE REVISED

Charles Kennedy RN, LNHA

I0475073

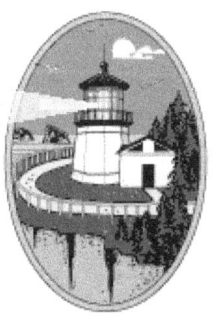

Lighthouse Senior Services
"Your Beacon for Solutions"

About the Author

Charles Kennedy RN, LNHA, CSSC.
Author, nurse and Founder of Lighthouse Senior Services. Has been a registered nurse since 1982. For almost 30 years his focus has been in geriatric care.
His work in both Skilled Nursing facilities as a Director of Nursing and Licensed Nursing Home Administrator. As well as a Director of Operations in the Home Health arena, has offered him the unique opportunity to understand the needs and frustrations of so many seniors and their loved ones.
Charles can be contacted at
kennedy@lighthouseseniorservices.com
Visit him at www.lighthouseseniorservices.com

CONTENTS

Introduction 5
Chapter 1   Residents Rights................. 9
Chapter 2   Take the Nursing LEAP........ 23
Chapter 3   Nursing Assessment............ 27
Chapter 4   Hot Rack Charting.............. 39
            Dialysis........................... 42
            Antibiotic Therapy............... 43
            Isolation.......................... 44
            Falls.............................. 45
            Gastro............................ 46
            IV Therapy....................... 47
            Genito/Urinary................... 48
            Medicare..........................49
            Musculoskeletal..................50
            Neurological..................... 51
            Psychiatric/Behavior............. 52
            Splint............................ 53
            Skin.............................. 54
            Respiratory....................... 55
            New Admit........................ 56
            Amputation....................... 57
            Anticoagulation.................. 58
            CHF.............................. 59
            CVA.............................. 60
            Diabetes......................... 61
            Fractured Hip.................... 62

	Tube Feeding....................	63
	Colostomy......................	64
	Pneumonia......................	65
	Seizure Disorder................	66
Chapter 5	HIPPA..........................	67
Chapter 6	Abuse...........................	73
Chapter 7	Infection Control...............	77
Chapter 8	Oxygen Therapy................	85
Chapter 9	Post Mortum Care..............	99
Chapter 10	Tips and Tricks.................	105
	Psych Tips......................	106
	Psych Meds.....................	108
	Bruising Guide..................	110
	Survey Preparation.............	115
	Reminders for Med Pass.......	117
	Hydration.......................	119
	Tube feeding and Medications	121
	Resident Aggression............	123
	Nursing Humor..................	132
	Common Lab Values............	134
	Signs and Symptoms of Chemical Imbalance...........	136
	Controlled Substances...........	138
	How to call a physician..........	140
	Things............................	143
	Abbreviations.....................151
	Common Medications...........	219

INTRODUCTION

Welcome to the world of Long Term Care. If you have been a LTC nurse for any length of time you know it is it's own world. Nurses in other arenas of healthcare never understand LTC till they are in it.

Nursing homes are the most regulated industry in the country, even more so than nuclear power plants. Because of the enormous amount of regulations and the fact that LTC is a cross between med-surg, home health and hospice. LTC nursing can be the most complex and challenging aspect of healthcare.

If you have ever had a hired worker in your house be it a handyman, plumber, or TV repairman, you know how you want them to respect your home, your privacy, and your belongings.

We are the handymen of healthcare. Every day we work in their home, their bedroom, and their dinning room.

We can never loose sight of this fact.

Even though we are there to help them, even though they may not have the cognition to know we are there, or there to help, we are working in their home.

As a director of nursing I always had a sign on my door that said

"I only have one rule and it's Golden"

Very often Staff feel that some others are beneath them. RN's are over LPN's, LPN's are over Cna's, and Cna's can talk down to a confused resident. Truth is regardless of who you are talking to, regardless of what they have done, treat them with the dignity and respect that you would want to be treated with yourself. I have terminated staff members for poor performance or unacceptable behavior and at the end of the meeting they smiled and thanked me for my time. All because I made it clear that I could not accept their actions but I accepted them as a person.

My suggestion to you, Have one rule and make it golden. Apply that rule to every person you come in contact with whereever you are in life. The road of life will be a lot less bumpy when you treat others with respect and you will be amazed at how contagious it can become.

Every facility has it's own set of policies and procedures. It is extremely important that you read the policies for your facility. They may do things

different from your last facility and the administration and public health will hold you to the policies where you are at. No one will listen to "We used to do it this way".
Be part of the new team.

This page blank

Chapter 1.
Resident Rights

Residents Rights

I am often asked, are resident rights really that important? No they are not that important.
THEY ARE EVEN MORE IMPORTANT.
Every aspect of the care you give can be traced back to resident rights.
As you read over the rights you will see they really are not just about residents but rather about human rights, the rights that every human being regard as basic. Being a resident in a nursing home does not mean they become second-class citizens.
It has been my experience that when residents and families are treated with respect, the whole process goes smoother and when issues do occur, everyone is much more understanding to the situation.

1. Your rights to safety and good care

Your facility must provide services to keep your physical and mental health, and sense of satisfaction with yourself, at their highest practical levels.

Your facility must be clean and stay at a healthy temperature.

You must not be abused by anyone — physically, verbally, mentally, financially or sexually.

Your facility must not physically restrain you unless there is no other way to keep you safe and you agree to the restraint.

You may be given medicine intended to change your mood or how you think *only with your permission* and only as part of an overall plan designed to change or remove the problems for which the medicines are given.

2. Your rights to participate in your own care

Your facility must develop a written care plan, which states all the services your facility will provide to you and everything you are expected to do. Your facility must make reasonable arrangements to meet your needs and choices.

You may go to the care plan conference where your care plan is decided.

You may choose to have family, friends or a representative participate in the care plan conference.

You have the right to choose your own doctor. You will have to pay the doctor yourself unless Medicare, your insurance plan or Medicaid will pay the doctor bill. -

Your facility must tell you the name and specialty of each doctor responsible for your care, and how to contact that doctor.

You have the right to be in charge of taking your own medicine if your care planning team and your doctor say that you are able to do so.

You have the right to refuse any medical treatment, if you refuse a treatment, your facility must tell you what may happen because of your refusal and tell you of other possible treatments. This is called a negotiated risk agreement and must be documented in your care plan.
You have the right to all information about your medical condition and treatment in a language that you can understand.

You have the right to make a Living Will or a *Durable Power of Attorney for Health Care,* so the facility will know your wishes if you can no longer speak for yourself.

You may refuse to participate in any experimental treatment or allow anyone to use information about you for research without your permission.

Your facility must allow you to see your medical records within 24 hours of your request. You may purchase a copy of part or all of your record at a reasonable copy fee with two working days' advance notice.

Your facility may not require you to work.
You have the right to move out of your facility after you give the administrator, nurse, or doctor written notice that you plan to move.

3. Your right to privacy

Your medical and personal care are private. Facility staff must respect your privacy when you are being examined or given care.

Facility staff must knock before entering your room.

Your facility may not give information about you or your care to unauthorized persons without your permission, unless you are being transferred to a hospital or to another health care facility.

You have the right to have private visits at a reasonable hour. The only exception is if your doctor has ordered limited visits for medical reasons.

You may ask any visitor to leave your personal living area at any time.

You have the right to make and receive phone calls in private.

Your facility must deliver your mail to you promptly, and promptly send mail out for you. Your facility may not open your mail.
If you are married, you and your spouse have the right to share a room unless no room is available or your doctor has said you cannot share a room for medical reasons.

4. Your rights regarding your money

You have the right to manage your own money. Without your written permission, your facility may not become your money manager or your Social Security representative payee.

If you ask your facility to manage your personal money for you, it must do so. (Medicare or Medicaid certified facilities only)
If your facility manages your money,
...it may spend your money only with your permission.
...it must give you an itemized written statement at least once every three months for all the money put into your account and all of the money taken out of your account.

..it must put your money in a bank account that earns interest for you if:
• you live in a Medicaid facility and have over $50 or
• you live in a licensed only facility and have over $100.

If your facility manages your money *and* you get Medicaid,
your facility must tell you if your savings come within $200 of the amount Medicaid allows you to keep. Money saved over that amount may be used to pay for your care in the facility. If you die, within 30 days of your death your facility must give your family, or whoever is in charge of distributing your property, a final accounting of all money left in any account that the facility managed for you.

You may see your financial record at any time

5. Your personal property rights

You have the right to keep and wear your own appropriate clothing.

You may keep and use your own property, including some furniture if there is enough space, unless this interferes with the health and safety of other residents.

You have the right to expect your facility to have a safe place where you can keep small valuables that you can get to daily.

Your facility must try to keep your property from being lost or stolen. If your property is missing, the facility must try to find it.

6. Your rights in paying for your care and getting Medicare and Medicaid

If you are paying for some or all of your care at your facility,
you must be given a contract that states what services are provided by the facility and how much they cost. The contract must say what expenses are not part of the regular rate.

Your facility must not require anyone else to sign an agreement saying that they will pay your bill if you cannot pay it yourself. The only one who can be required to pay your bill for you is a court appointed guardian or someone else who is handling your money for you.

Your facility must give you information about how to apply for Medicaid and Medicare and rules about "spousal impoverishment." Spousal impoverishment rules allow you to give money and property to your spouse and still be eligible for Medicaid.

You have the right to apply for Medicaid or Medicare to help pay for your care.
If you receive Medicaid, the facility may not make you pay for anything for which Medicaid pays. The facility must give you a written list of what items and services Medicaid pays, and items and services for which you could be charged.

7. Your rights to stay in your facility

You have the right to keep living in your facility, unless your facility forces you to move because you are dangerous to yourself or others, your medical needs cannot be met, you have not paid or are late paying your bill, or your facility closes.

You must be given written notice *(Notice of Involuntary Transfer or Discharge Pursuant to the Nursing Home Care Act)* within 21 days of the departure date, if your facility requests you to move from the facility. If you do not receive the written notice, ask for it. By moving and not receiving the notice, you may be agreeing to a voluntary transfer to another residence.

If requested, the notice must:

tell you why your facility wants you to move,

tell you how you can file an appeal to the Department

 of Public Health and include a stamped, addressed

envelope for you to mail your appeal to the Department of Public Health.
You have the right to appeal to the Department of Public Health. If you choose to appeal:

A health hearing officer will travel to your facility to hear you tell why you believe you should stay in the facility and why the facility believes you
should move.

The facility cannot make you leave until the appeal is decided by the Department of Public Health.

Help is available with your appeal. Contact your Long Term Care Ombudsman for help in appealing your involuntary transfer or discharge.

If you have a developmental disability or mental illness, you may ask Equip for Equality for help in appealing your involuntary transfer or discharge.

Before your facility can transfer or discharge you, it must prepare and orient you to be sure that your discharge is safe and that you will be moving to an appropriate setting.

You must be allowed to return to your facility after you are hospitalized, unless your facility gives you written notice as described above.
If you receive Medicaid and are hospitalized for 10 or fewer days, your facility must let you return

when you leave the hospital even if the facility has given you a Notice of Involuntary Transfer or Discharge.

If you are hospitalized for more than 10 days, your facility must let you return if it has a bed available and you still need that kind of care.
If your facility is full, you must be allowed to have the first available semi-private room, if you still need that kind of care.

You have the right to be told in advance if your room or roommate is being changed. (Medicare or Medicaid certified facilities only)

8. Your rights as a citizen and a facility resident

Your facility must let you see reports of all inspections by the Illinois Department of Public Health from the last five years and the most recent survey of your facility along with any corrective action plans from your facility.

You do not lose your rights as a citizen of your state and the United States because you live in a long term care facility.

If a court of law has appointed a legal guardian for you, your guardian may exercise your rights for you, according to the court order.

If you have named an agent under a Durable Power of Attorney for Health Care, your agent may exercise your rights for you.

You have freedom of religion. At your request, the facility must make arrangements for you to attend religious services of your choice as long as you agree to pay any travel-related costs. The facility may not force you to follow any religious beliefs or practices and cannot require you to attend any religious services.

You have the right to vote for the candidate of your choice in public elections.

You have the right to participate in social and community activities that do not interfere with the rights of other residents.

You have the right to participate with other residents in the Resident council. Your facility must respond to concerns raised by the council.

You have the right to meet with the Long Term Care Ombudsman, community organizations, social service groups, legal advocates, and members of the general public who come to your facility.

Representatives of these groups may come to your facility to provide services, tell you about your rights, or help you assert your rights.

You have the right to present grievances...

to your facility and to get a prompt response. Your facility may not threaten or punish you in any way for asserting your rights or presenting grievances. to outside organizations and advocates including the
following agencies:
Long Term Care Ombudsman:

This page blank

Chapter 2
The Nursing L.E.A.P.

Take the NURSING L.E.A.P

That is to say Accept the following

Leadership,
Excellence,
Accountability,
Pride.

Leadership

Take Charge of your unit. CNA's report to you.
The nurse NOT the CNA make out the
assignments.
The nurse is responsible to frequently make
rounds to follow up on CNA's to ensure that
residents are dressed, up, clean, dry, and safe.
Monitor that showers, nails, hair, shaves are done.
The Nurse is to oversee total care of a resident.
Supervise your team to include; residents, showers,
toileting, breaks/lunch times, use of gait belts,
proper use of hoyer, and sit-to-stand.

Excellence

Promote Quality of care at all levels. Double-check your own work for error free delivery, Develop a sense of ownership with your residents, unit, and staff.

Practice the "One rule that's golden" philosophy. Recognize that we cannot control all events. But we can control our reaction to those events.

Accountability

Accept responsibility for your team.

Follow thru on orders, Admissions,T.O.'s, P.O.S's, Mar's, Tar's, Test Req's, Test center Transportation. Follow up on medications

Fax orders in a timely manner.

Check on delivery. Monitor for re-orders. Utilize "C" and "E" box appropriately.

Follow up on tests; Obtain order, Complete req, Contact test facility, Arrange for any necessary transportation.

Obtain timely results

Notify MD of results

Process any new orders.

Complete necessary documentation

Utilize HOT RACK CHARTING.

Hot Rack charting is the Proper use of 24hour report,

Appropriate behavior charting, Correct use of the incident report. Complete MAR's, Tar's, behavior sheets. Complete wound and skin sheets
Proper MD and family notification of any significant change.

Pride

Care about how your team reflects on you.
Care how your unit looks.
Care how your residents look, sound, or smell.
Care how your staff presents themselves to residents, families, or guests. Become the resident's advocate at every level.

Chapter 3
Resident Assessments

RESIDENT ASSESSMENT

1. INSPECTION: The process of examining the surface of the body and it is movements utilizing visual, auditory and olfactory senses for gathering information. Inspection should be purposeful and systematic comparing bilateral body parts, and continues throughout the entire examination.

2. PALPATION: The technique of using touch to gather information about temperature, turgor. texture, moisture, vibrations, and shape. May use light palpation, which is the application of pressure by closed fingers and depressing the skin and underlying structures about 1.3 inch, or deep palpation, using inward pressure to about I inch. The client should be provided with privacy, the nurse should have warm hands with short fingernails, and the area of tenderness should be palpated last
.

3. PERCUSSION: The art of striking one object with another to create sound, so that one can assess the location, size and density of underlying tissues. The no dominant hand is placed on the area to be percussed with fingers slightly separated and the dommant hand is used as the sinking force by exerting a sharp downward wrist movement so that the tip of the middle finger on the dominant hand strikes the joint of the middle finger on the non-dominant hand.

The five percussion tones are

tympany - loud drumlike sound
resonance - moderate to loud, low-pitch, hollow sound
hyper resonance - very loud, low-pitch, booming sound
flatness -soft, high-pitch, flat sound
dullness - soft to moderate, high-pitch, thud-like sound

4. AUSCULTATION

The act of listening to sounds produced by the body using a stethoscope. The stethoscope has a diaphragm that detects high-pitched sounds best and a bell that detects low-pitched sounds best.

Four characteristics of sound should be noted
Pitch, loudness, Quality, Duration

There are three normal breath sounds.
(B)   Bronchial breath sounds-*loud, harsh, high pitched.* Heard over trachea, bronchi (between clavicles and midsternum), and over main bronchus.

(BV) Bronchovesicular breath sounds-blowing sounds, moderate intensity and pitch.
Heard over large airways, on either side of sternum, at the Angle of Louis, and between scapulae.
(V)Vesicular breath sounds- Soft breezy quality, low pitched.

Abnormal Lung Sounds

SOUND	CHARACTERISTICS	LUNG PROBLEM
Crackles	popping, crackling, bubbling, moist sounds on inspiration	pneumonia, pulmonary edema, pulmonary fibrosis
Rhonchi	rumbling sound on expiration	pneumonia, emphysema, bronchitis, bronchiectasis
Wheezes	high-pitched musical sound during both inspiration and expiration (louder)	emphysema, asthma, foreign bodies

The 5 P's of circulatory checks

Pain –
Pallor –
Paralysis –
Paresthesia –
Pulse

EDEMA

Assess by placing a finger over the dorsum of the foot or tiba for 5 seconds

0	No edema
1+	Barely discernible depression
2+	A deeper depression (less than 5 mm) accompanied by normal foot and leg contours
3+	Deep depression (5 to 10 mm) accompanied by foot and leg swelling
4+	An even deeper depression (more than 1 cm) accompanied by severe foot and leg swelling

Pedal Pulses

Peripheral pulses should be compared for rate, rhythm, and quality.

Pulses are graded as follows.

0 Absent –
+1 Weak and thready –
+2 Normal –
+3 Full –
+4 Bounding

Grading of Heart Murmurs

Grade I Faint; heard after nurse has concentrated
Grade II Faint murmur heard immediately
Grade III Moderately loud, not associated with thrill
Grade IV Loud and may be associated with a thrill
Grade V Very loud; associated with thrill
Grade VI Very loud; heard with stethoscope off chest, associated with thrill

Heart Sounds

S1

The first heart sound - S1 - is in time with the pulse in your carotid artery in your neck. The sound of the tricuspid valve closing may be louder in patients with pulmonary hypertension due to increased pressure beyond the valve. Non-heart-related factors such as obesity, muscularity, emphysema, and fluid around the heart can reduce both S1 and S2.

The position of the valves when the ventricles contract can have a big effect on the first heart sound. If the valves are wide open when the ventricule contracts, a loud S1 is heard. This can occur with anemia, fever or hyperthyroid.

When the valves are partly closed when the ventricule contracts, S1 is faint. Beta-blockers produce a fainter S1. Structural changes in the heart valves can also affect S1. Fibrosis and calcification of the mitral valve may reduce S1, while stenosis of the mitral valve may cause a louder S1.

S2

The second heart sound marks the beginning of diastole - the heart's relaxation phase - when the ventricles fill with blood. In children and teenagers, S2 may be more pronounced. Right ventricular ejection time is slightly longer than left ventricular ejection time. As a result, the pulmonic valve closes a little later than the aortic valve.

Higher closing pressures occur in patients with chronic high blood pressure, pulmonary hypertension, or during exercise or excitement. This results in a louder A2 (the closing sound of the aortic valve).

On the other hand, low blood pressure reduces the sound. The second heart sound may be "split" in patients with right bundle branch block, which results in delayed pulmonic valve closing. Left bundle branch block may cause aortic valve closing (A2) to be slower than pulmonic valve closing (P2).

S3

During diastole there are 2 sounds of ventricular filling: The first is from the atrial walls and the second is from the contraction of the atriums. The third heart sound is caused by vibration of the ventricular walls, resulting from the first rapid filling so it is heard just after S2. The third heart sound is low in frequency and intensity. An S3 is commonly heard in children and young adults. In older adults and the elderly with heart disease, an S3 often means heart failure.

S4

The fourth heart sound occurs during the second phase of ventricular filling: when the atriums contract just before S1. As with S3, the fourth heart sound is thought to be caused by the vibration of valves, supporting structures, and the

ventricular walls. An abnormal S4 is heard in
people with conditions that increase resistance to
ventricular filling, such as a weak left ventricle.

Other Abnormal Heart Sounds

opening snap
is caused by a noncompliant valve, such as a mitral
valve in a patient with a history of rheumatic fever
ejection click
is a high-pitched sound occurring shortly after S1.
It is associated with a dilated pulmonary artery or
septal defects
pericardial friction rub
is a to-and-fro sound that waxes and wanes with
diastole and systole. It is present even when the
patient holds his breath
murmur
is a vague sound associated with turbulent blood
flow through a heart valve. Turbulent blood flow
may be the result of:
increased flow across a normal valve
forward flow across an irregular or constricted
valve, or into an enlarged heart chamber
back-flow through an insufficient valve

thrill
is a vibration, high in frequency and sustained. If a
vibration is felt but no murmur is heard, the
vibration is not called a thrill

pericardial knock
is a high-pitched sound best heard during diastole.
Pericardial knocks are caused by a thick
pericardium limiting expansion of the ventricle
during the filling phase (diastole)

The Third Heart Sound - S3

A third heart sound may be the earliest clue to
heart failure. It predicts a high risk of
complications in non-heart surgery. CHF patients
with an S3 will probably respond well to digoxin.
However, detecting S3 is inconsistent even among
experienced doctors. While an S3 may have
important implications for treatment, many doctors
cannot detect it. The following is some history and
the current thinking on heart sounds and their
usefulness.

In 1856, Potain first described "gallop rhythm"
as a tripling or quadrupling of heart sounds
sounding like the canter of a horse. That term is
still used to describe a third or fourth heart sound.
Gallops are diastolic events - they occur during the
heart's relaxation phase, when it fills with blood.
S3 seems to be related to the filling phase and S4
seems to be related to atrial contraction.

S3 is well recognized as an early clue to the
presence of heart disease. S3 may offer valuable
information about diagnosis, prognosis, and
treatment. It occurs 0.12 to 0.16 seconds after the

second heart sound. Potain suggested that S3 results from the sudden stop of the ventricle's expansion as it fills with blood. It is agreed that S3 is associated with over-expansion of the ventricle during the filling phase.

Coulshed and Epstein return to the original theory: "Our evidence supports the original concept that S3 occurs when the rapidly filling ventricle reaches a point when its expansion is halted by the resistance of its wall. The resulting vibrations are heard as the third heart sound." Pozzoli confirmed that the rapid slowing of the left ventricle at the end of filling is the most likely cause of S3.

As the rush of blood into the heart's ventricles during filling comes to a sudden halt - when it reaches maximum filling - the kinetic energy of the blood's movement is converted to vibration. These vibrations can sometimes be heard. The higher the inflow rate and the higher the filling rate, the greater the blood's deceleration, and the more likely an S3 will occur.

S3 in young adults may be explained by the relatively large motion of the heart and the thin chest wall. S3 disappears around age 40 in healthy people.

Detecting Heart Sounds

To detect heart sounds, the patient should be lying down and examined in a quiet room. Left-sided S3 is best heard at the apex of the heart (the lower pointed end of the heart) with the patient lying on his left side. It is a low-pitched sound and heard best using the bell of the stethoscope with light pressure. It follows the second heart sound in timing. S4 is more easily heard after mild exertion in the presence of a fast heart rate, and also with the legs elevated.

Things that usually prevent S3 detection are surrounding noise, obesity, emphysema, failure to use the stethescope properly, and examining the patient in a seated position. Simple maneuvers like closing the door to the exam room to reduce surrounding noise helps in detecting S3.

If heart rate is higher than 100 beats per minute, finding third and fourth heart sounds is impossible. Unless the heart rate is slowed, the examiner can only guess at telling S3 from S4 unless there is a-fib, which eliminates the possibility of an S4.

Chapter 4
HOT RACK CHARTING

HOT RACK CHARTING

All Residents who are on the 24 Hour Report will need documentation in the nurse's notes each shift using the following guidelines. Hot rack charts are to include but are not limited to:

1.   New admits and Readmits for 72 hours (9 shifts total), including vital signs.
2.   Incident reports for 72 hours (9 shifts total) after the incident.
3.   Residents on antibiotics for the duration of the antibiotic therapy and for 72 hours following completion of the antibiotic.
4.   IV Therapy
5.   Residents who have experienced a change in condition (i.e. vomiting or diarrhea, congested, febrile, initial identification of a pressure ulcer, etc.)
6.   All Medicare residents
7.   Residents on Isolation

It is the responsibility of the nurse to utilize these guidelines and complete thorough documentation in the nurse's notes.

General Guidelines

DO NOT BLOCK CHART

ALL ENTRIES IN THE CHART MUST HAVE A DATE AND TIME

THE TIME MUST CORRESPOND TO THE EVENT NOT EVERYTHING YOU DID IN THE LAST 45 MINUTES

Example:

08:10 Found resident un responsive

08:11 vital signs absent CPR initiated

08:13 Cna called 911

The following are minimum requirements for each type of condition, disease or event.

DIALYSIS

1. Complete set of Vital Signs
2. Day of last dialysis
3. Monitoring for adverse reactions
4. Skin/rashes noted
5. Condition of access
6. Lab Results, culture and screening, UA, etc
7. Fluids offered, appetite

ANTIBIOTIC THERAPY

1. Temperature
2. Type of Antibiotic Resident is using
3. Monitoring for adverse reactions
4. Skin/rashes noted
5. Reason that ABT is required
6. Lab Results, culture and screening, UA, etc
7. Fluids offered, appetite

ISOLATION

1. Complete set of Vital Signs
2. Type of Isolation and "Isolation Maintained"
3. AST, if any
4. Location of Infection
5. Turning and Repositioning for Bed ridden Residents
6. Appetite
7. Fluids offered

FALLS

1. Complete Vital Signs
2. Pain, type and location, intensity
3. Range of Motion
4. Edema, deformity
5. Weight bearing and activity
6. Skin status, i.e. hematomas, bruising, skin tears, lacerations, reddened areas,
7. Level of Consciousness,
8. Neuros, Orientation to time, place and person, pupil responses, strength of extremities,
9. Headache nausea & vomiting
10. Physician notification
11. family notification
12. Any treatments and or nursing Interventions utilized
13. Time of calling for transportation and expected ETA of transport
14. Time that the Resident was picked up by Ambulance

GASTROINTESTINAL

1. Complete set of Vital Signs
2. Nausea, vomiting, flatulence, bowel sounds
3. Appitite, difficult swallowing
4. Character, color, frequency of stools, date of last BM
5. Rectal conditions, bleeding, fistulas, hemorrhoids
6. Check for fecal impaction
7. Distention
8. Pain type and location,Rating
9. Physician notified
10. Family notified
11. Any treatment or medical or nursing intervention such as rectal tube, diet or medication change

IV THERAPY

1. Complete set of Vital Signs
2. Type of IV Fluids
3. Rate of Fluid
4. Intake & Output
5. IV Site monitored for infiltration and phlebitis
6. Lung sounds
7. Additives or Medications given per IV

GENITOURINARY

1. Complete set of Vital Signs
2. Pain type and location, Pain Rating
3. Urine Color, Odor, Amounts, Clarity
4. Micturation (Urgency, Hesitancy, Dysuria, incontinence, frequency)
5. Intake and Output
6. Urinary retention/Abdominal Distention
7. Level of Consciousness
8. Behavioral Changes
9. Physician Notification
10. Family notification
11. Any Treatments or medical nursing interventions that are taken such as lab tests, catheterization, etc

MEDICARE RESIDENTS

1. Complete set of Vital Signs
2. Pain type and location, if any, as well as pain rating
3. Lung sounds
4. Bowel sounds
5. Pedal pulses, CMS
6. Skin assessment
7. Appetite
8. Fluids offered and taken PT, OT, ST as well as # of days per week that the Resident is seen by therapy
10. Orientation to time, person, and place
11. Mobility/Activity level and tolerance
12. Any treatments and nursing/medical interventions that are taken

MUSCULOSKELETAL

1. Complete set of vital signs
2. Pain type and location, Pain Rating
3. Strength or weakness
4. Edema/Deformity/Range of Motion/Weight bearing
5. Hematoma or eccymosis
6. Physician Notification
7. Family Notification
8. Any treatments or medical/nursing interventions that are taken such as use of w/c, trapeze, PT, walker, etc

NEUROLOGICAL

1. Complete set of Vital signs
2. Pain type and location, Pain Rating
3. Level of Consciousness /dizziness / memory
4. Seizures including length of the seizure and post ictal condition
5. Movement and Strength of extremities
6. Orientation to time, person and place
7. Pupil Responses headaches nausea and vomiting
8. Sleep patterns
9. Speech paterns
10. Physician notified
11. Family Notification

PSYCHOLOGICAL BEHAVIORS

1. Specific Behavioral Changes Use quotes and describe actual behaviors exhibited
2. Hallucinations
3. Physician Notification
4. Family Notification
5. Affect and interaction with others
6. Any Treatment or Medical/nursing interventions that are taken such as behavior management, medications given, redirection, etc.
7. Psychotropic Medications used and Monitored for effect and tolerance

SPLINT CARE

1. Peripheral Circulation (Distal pulses, color, capillary refill, temperature of extremity)
2. Edema/paresthesia
3. Skin status (odor, drainage, color, open areas)
4. Pain type and location, Pain rating
5. Condition of Cast
6. Weight bearing/Strength of extremity
7. Activity level
8. Physician Notification
9. Family Notification
10. Any treatment or medical/nursing interventions taken such as elevation, splints, use of assistive device.

SKIN

1. Complete Vital Signs
2. Location of Abnormality
3. Precise measurements and Stage of Wound
4. Color
5. Drainage amount, type odor and color
6. Mobility status / activity level
7. Body Weight and alterations
8. Continence
9. Nutritional status
10. Prevention methods utilized Such as Turning and positioning, Skin Care rendered, Creams and Ointments (Proshield or Soothe & Cool),
11. Special mattress, w/c Gel pads.
12. Inflammation or Edema
13. Impairments of circulation, neurological, musculoskeletal, immune system, etc.
14. Any treatments or medical/nursing interventions that are taken such as medications (sedatives, imrnunosuppressant, steroids, ABT), Splints, Prosthesis, Catheters
15. Physician Notification
16. Family Notification

RESPIRATORY
1. Complete set of Vital Signs
2. Shortness of Breath
3. Pain type and location, pain
4. Bilateral Lung Sounds
5. Pulse Oximetry (O2 Sats)
6. Color of skin, especially nail beds and mucosa
7. Tracheobronchial secretions, amount and character
8. Use of accessory muscles for breathing
9. Abnormal Breathing patterns
    (Apnea, Cheyne-Stokes, Tachypnea)
10. Physician Notification
11 .Family Notification

Any treatment or medical /nursing interventions that are taken, such as oxygen, suction, labwork, High Fowlers position, nebulizer treatments, etc.

NEW ADMISSIONS / READMISSIONS

1. Complete set of Vital Signs
2. Skin Assessment on Admission Form
3. Monitor Conditions noted on Admission assessment
4. Mental Status
5. Appetite
6. Activity Tolerance and limitations
7. Bowel and Bladder habits
8. Abnormalities not noted on admission assessments
9. Monitoring of Medications and Resident response
10. Any treatments or medical nursing interventions
11. Accurate height and weight
12. NOTE: Admission packet must be completed during the first shift that the Resident is admitted/readmitted. This includes:
    -Bowel and Bladder assessment
    -Pneumonia Assessment
    -Fall Risk Assessment
    -Side Rail Assessment
    -Pressure Ulcer Risk Assessment
    -Pain Assessment
    -Dehydration
    -Foley (Only if Resident has an Indwelling Foley) Must have a diagnosis or D/C order for all foley admissions

AMPUTATION

1. Vital signs
2. Open Wound
   a. treatment and frequency
   b. wound size, drainage, amount of
   c. discharge, color, and odor
   d. edema (check every shift)
3. Circulatory checks (every shift)
   a. motion
   b. sensation
   c. circulation
4. Application and progress of stump shrinker
5. Development of contractures
6. Presence of callus formations
7. Check unaffected foot for foot drop
8. Note "phantom" pain
   a. where
   b. when
   c. type
   d. duration
   e. how treated
   f. results of treatment
9. Balance, standing and sitting
10. Note ambulation progress
11. Prosthetic Device (note skin condition under device)
12. Problems with body image
13. Participation hi PT/OT programs
14. Tolerance of prosthetic device

<u>ANTICOAGULATION THERAPY</u>

1.) Vital signs
2.) Pain (bone, abdominal, joint or other pain)
3.) Presence or absence of active bleeding.
   a. hematuria
   b. petechiae
   c. bruising
   d. bloody stools
   e. nose bleeds
   f. bloody gums
4.) Presence or absence of signs of hemorrhage under the skin. (oral mucosa, conjunctiva)
5.) Results of pro-times or PTTs
6.) Color (cyanosis or pallor)
7.) Document teaching of signs and symptoms of anti coagulant complications
8.) Communication with physician and family

CONGESTIVE HEART FAILURE

1.) Complete vital signs (apical heart rate)
2.) Irregularities in vital signs
2.) Auscultation of lungs (presence of rales, wheezing, and congestion)
4.) Edema (1+ - 4+ every shift)
5.) Diuretic therapy - response, intake & output
6.) Use of oxygen (rate, how often)
7.) Dyspnea or SOB
8.) Chest pain, action taken and resident's response
9.) Mobility (ambulation status)
10.) Weakness
11.) HOB elevated
12.) Daily weight if ordered
13.) Communication with MD and family

CVA (RIGHT OR LEFT)

1.) Vital Signs
2.) Documentassistance needed for ADLs
3.) Document amount of assistance needed for bed mobility, positioning and transfers
4.) Document problems with balance and how it affects level of functioning
5.) Document safety measures needed
6.) Edema of affected side
7.) Speech involvement - able to make needs known
8.) Restorative program
   a. feeding
   b. bowel and bladder
   c. appliance if required (sling or splint)
9.) document skin condition under appliance
10.) Swallowing problems:
   a, drooling
   b. choking
   c. coughing
   d. pocketing of food in his mouth
11.) Changes in condition
12.) Equipment necessary (wheelchair, walker, trapeze)
13.) Contractures (preventative)
14.) PT, OT and ST participation
15.) Physician notification

DIABETES MELLITUS - INSULIN DEPENDENT RESIDENT UNABLE TO ADMINISTER OWN INSULIN

1.) Vital signs
2.) Diet - intake – appetite
3.) Signs and symptoms of hypo/hyperglycemic reaction (action taken and residents response)
4.) BGM (frequency and results) sliding scale dose given if needed.
5.) Signs of infection
6.) Lab work (notified MD)
7.) Skin care
8.) Reason resident unable to administer own insulin (weekly note)
9.) Physician notification

FRACTURED HIP

1.) Complete vital signs
5.) Pain (frequency, amount)
6.) Suture line (describe in detail, redness, sutures, drainage, odor)
7.) Mobility (document assistance needed for bed mobility
8.) Transfer (document assistance needed to transfer and assist required to <u>maintain</u> weight bearing status)
9.) Circulation checks
10.) Document degree of assistance needed in ADLs and endurance level.
11.) Weight bearing status
12.) Mental status (ability to cooperate)
13.) Edema of affected extremity
14.) Equipment needed (w/c walker)
15.) PT and OT program - residents Response
16.) Physician Notification

Tube Feeding

1.) Vital signs
2.) Feeding schedule (bolus, gravity or pump, how often and how much)
3.) Daily caloric intake
4.) Feeding formula
5.) Checking position of tube (i.e., auscultating abdomen after injecting air)
6.) Dressings present and how often changed (describe any drainage and surrounding skin condition)
7.) Weight
8.) Intake and output
9.) Complications of feeding (IE diarrhea, vomiting)
10.) Number, size of feeding tube
11.) Frequency of flush and amount
12.) HOB elevated (degrees)
13.) Level of consciousness
14.) Medications given via tube
15.) Swallowing ability (speech therapy consultation)
16.) Resident's tolerance to feeding

COLOSTOMY / ILEOSTOMY

1.) Vital signs
2.) Observation of ostomy site
   a. reddness
   b. purulent drainage
   c. open areas
   d. skin condition around stoma
   e. color and size of stoma
3.) Stool: frequency, consistency, amount, and color
4.) Abdominal Distention: bowel sounds
5.) Irrigations: solution, frequency, and results
6.) Teaching progress
   a. what tasks have been taught
   b. assess resident's learning ability
   c. return demonstration
7.) Appliance used
8.) Additional skin care needed
9.) Physician Notification

PNEUMONIA

1.) Complete vital signs
   a. temperature increases or decreases
   b. fever
   c. chills
2.) Auscultation of lungs (presence of rales, congestion)
3.) Cough (painful, hacking, productive, nonproductive)
4.) Sputum (describe amt and color)
5.) Ability to cough and deep breath
6.) Color (flushed face, cyanosis or pallor)
7.) Dyspnea
8.) Nutritional status / hydration status
9.) Intake and output
10.) Immobility and weakness (Is resident ambulatory or bed ridden? Is he able to change position in bed by self?)
11.) Frequent changes in position
12.) Oxygen therapy (liter flow, type used, how often)
13.) Endurance level with activity
14.) Suctioning
15.) Mental status changes
16.) Physician Notification and family

SEIZURE DISORDER
1.) Complete vital signs (post seizure)
2.) Time began
3.) Duration
4.) Symptoms at beginning
5.) Type (grand mal petit)
6.) Type of movements\
7.) Unconsciousness (check airway)
8.) Incontinence
9.) Size of pupils
10.) Injuries sustained during seizure
11.) Medication
12.) Exhaustion (sleeping afterward)
13.) Therapeutic / diagnostic procedures
14.) Equipment (padded tongue blade, airway, padded side rails)
15.) Physician and family notified

Chapter 5
HIPPA

CONFIDENTIAL INFORMATION

Medical and other personal information regarding residents of the facility must be protected in order to respect the privacy of each resident and fulfill legal obligations of the facility and its professional staff. In addition, general information regarding resident care at the facility is confidential and may not be disclosed to the public
Employees must not discuss any medical nursing or other confidential information of any type with any person, unless it is necessary to carry out the employee's job duties. Communication of necessary information should be carried out in a discreet manner and not in a loud voice that others can overhear.

The U.S. Department of Health and Human Services (HHS) enforces the Federal privacy regulations commonly known as the **HIPAA Privacy Rule (HIPAA)**. HIPAA requires most doctors, nurses, pharmacies, hospitals, nursing homes, and other health care providers to protect the privacy of your health information. Here is a list of common questions about HIPAA and when health care providers may discuss or share your health information with your family members, friends, or others involved in your care or payment for care.

COMMON QUESTIONS ABOUT HIPAA

1. If I do not object, can my health care provider share or discuss my health information with my family, friends, or others involved in my care or payment for my care?

Yes. As long as you do not object, your health care provider is allowed to share or discuss your health information with your family, friends, or others involved in your care or payment for your care. Your provider may ask your permission, may tell you he or she plans to discuss the information and give you an opportunity to object, or may decide, using his or her professional judgment, that you do not object. In any of these cases, your health care provider may discuss only the information that the person involved needs to know about your care or payment for your care. Here are some examples: • An emergency room doctor may discuss your treatment in front of your friend when you ask that your friend come into the treatment room. • Your hospital may discuss your bill with your daughter who is with you at the hospital and has questions about the charges. • Your doctor may talk to your sister who is driving you home from the hospital about your keeping your foot raised during the ride home. • Your doctor may discuss the drugs you need to take with your health aide who has come with you to your appointment. • Your nurse may tell you that she is going to tell your brother how you are doing, and then she may discuss your health status with your brother if you did not say that she should not.

BUT: • Your nurse may not discuss your condition with your brother if you tell her not to.

2. **If I am unconscious or not around, can my health care provider still share or discuss my health information with my family, friends, or others involved in my care or payment for my care?** Yes. If you are not around or cannot give permission, your health care provider may share or discuss your health information with family, friends, or others involved in your care or payment for your care if he or she believes, in his or her professional judgment, that it is in your best interest. When someone other than a friend or family member is asking about you, your health care provider must be reasonably sure that you asked the person to be involved in your care or payment for your care. Your health care provider may share your information face to face, over the phone, or in writing, but may only share the information that the family

member, friend, or other person needs to know about your care or payment for your care. Here are some examples: • A surgeon who did emergency surgery on you may tell your spouse about your condition, either in person or by phone, while you are unconscious. • A pharmacist may give your prescription to a friend you send to pick it up. • A doctor may discuss your drugs with your caregiver who calls your doctor with a question about the right dosage. BUT: • A nurse may not tell your friend about a past medical problem that is unrelated to your current condition.

3. **Do I have to give my health care provider written permission to share or discuss my health information with my family members, friends, or others involved in my care or payment for my care?** HIPAA does not require that you give your health care provider written permission. However, your provider may prefer or require that you give written permission.

4. **If my family or friends call my health care provider to ask about my condition, will they have to give my provider proof of who they are?** HIPAA does not require proof of identity in these cases. However, your health care provider may have his or her own rules for verifying who is on the phone.

5. **Can I have another person pick up my prescription drugs, medical supplies, or X-rays?** Yes. HIPAA allows health care providers (such as pharmacists) to give prescription drugs, medical supplies, X-rays, and other health care items to a family member, friend, or other person you send to pick them up.

6. **Can my health care provider discuss my health information with an interpreter?** Yes. HIPAA allows your health care provider to share your health information with an interpreter who works for the provider to help communicate with you or your family, friends, or others involved in your care. If the interpreter is someone who does not work for your health care provider, HIPAA also allows your provider to discuss your health information with the interpreter so long as you do not object.

Chapter 6
Abuse and abuse reporting

Abuse Reporting

ABUSE/THREATS

The term "abuse" means any physical or mental injury or sexual assault inflicted on a person other than accidental means. Abuse of anv nature will not be tolerated. Any suspected abuse of a resident or other person must be reported to the Nursing Supervisor/Department Head immediately. The Nursing Supervisor/Department Head must immediately notify the Administrator.

The serious nature of an allegation of resident abuse sometimes requires that employees be suspended or reassigned pending the outcome of the investigation of those allegations. Any suspension or reassignment of this type is precautionary only and is not a disciplinary action intended to reflect adversely on the employee. Depending on the nature of the incident, or if any person is viewed as an immediate danger to residents, visitors, or staff, the police will be called immediately to intervene. Any documented occurrences will be reported to the Department of Public Health for follow-up investigation.

EXAMPLES
Hitting
Restraining a Resident without justification
Leaving a resident in need
Swearing at a resident
Degrading a resident
Threatening a resident
Withholding food or water
Refusing care
Teaching them a lesson
Mocking
Scolding
Patronizing attitude
Inappropriate touching
Sexual Harassment
Theft
Sexual Assault

TRIGGER WORDS
"Abuse"
"Hit/Slapped"
"Threatened me"
"He/She Hurt Me"
"Rape"
"Inappropriate"
"Scared"

WHAT NEEDS TO BE DONE WHEN YOU SUSPECT POSSIBLE ABUSE

Report It Immediately To the Administrator or your Supervisor Any allegation

 Regardless of whether you believe it

Regardless of whether you think the report is wrong.

Offenders can be anyone staff, another resident or even a visitor or family member

Cooperate in the investigation!

Chapter 7
Infection Control

Contact Precautions

need to be used for the following infections:

MRSA
VRE
ESBL
C-Diff

If your resident has a culture with one of these organisms, you must use contact precautions.
If you are treating the resident for Scabies (Elimite or <u>Stromectol),</u> the resident must be isolated from the time of the order, until the shower in the morning. The room is to be disinfected no matter which treatment is used.

Methicillin Resistant Staphylococcus Aureus

(MRSA) are particular strains of common bacteria which have developed resistance to all penicillins, including the usually effective methicillin and oxacillin. These strains are also resistant to cephalosporins, and thus present a serious epidemiologic challenge, especially in the long term care environments. of individuals affected by MRSA.

MRSA Infection –

Clinical symptoms present: fever, elevated WBC, productive cough with purulent sputum (if respiratory tract infection); OR, purulent drainage/ redness, infiltration, WBCs present. in the direct smear (if wound is present).
Positive culture for MRSA

MRSA Collonization

No clinical symptoms: Normal level of WBC, no productive cough; OR, no drainage or serious drainage (if open Wound) stable clinical status.

Positive culture for MRSA
(wounds, nares, perineum, anus
urine - infection site dependent)

ESBL

ESBL stands for Extended Spectrum Beta-Lactamase. A Beta-Lactamase is an enzyme produced by a bacteria which breaks down certain types of antibiotics.
ESBL producing bacteria are resistant to some of the antibiotics used to treat infection when it occurs. This resistance makes infection more difficult to treat.
Infection from ESBL producing bacteria occurs mainly in urine, but also may infect wounds & the

blood. Sometimes these bacteria can be in your body (usually your gut) but not make you unwell. This is called colonization instead of infection, as you feel well with no signs or symptoms of infection.

Clostridium difficile

C. difficile is a spore forming bacteria which can be part of the normal intestinal flora. C. difficile is the major cause of pseudomembranous colitis and antibiotic associated diarrhea.

C. difficile-associated disease occurs when the normal intestinal flora is altered, allowing C. difficile to flourish in the intestinal tract and produce a toxin that causes a watery diarrhea. Repeated enemas, prolonged nasogastric tube insertion and gastrointestinal tract surgery increase a person's risk of developing the disease. The overuse of antibiotics, especially penicillin (ampicillin), clindamycin and ephalosporins may also alter the normal intestinal flora and increase the risk of developing C. difficile diarrhea.

ISOLATION CULTURE GUIDELINES

MRSA
2 Negative results obtained 24 hours apart
48hours after antibiotic completed.

ESBL and VRE
3 Negative results obtained 1 week apart,
1 week after antibiotic completed.

C-DIFF
2 Negative results obtained 1 week apart,
1 week after antibiotic completed.
Some MDs want three.

INFLUENZA AND PNEUMONIA

- Influenza (FLU) is a serious disease of the nose, throat, and lungs that is caused by influenza viruses. Influenza can lead to pneumonia. It can cause mild to severe illness, and at times can lead to death.
The best way to prevent the flu is by getting a flu vaccine each year.
Symptoms of the FLU
    High Fever
    Headache
    Extreme tiredness
    Dry cough
    Sore throat
    Runny or stuffy nose
    Muscle aches

Complications: Bacterial Pneumonia, ear infections, sinus infections, dehydration, worsening of Chronic conditions such as Congestive Heart Failure, Asthma, and Diabetes. How It Spreads:
Coughing, Sneezing by people who have the flu.

Touching something with the flu virus on it and then touching your mouth or nose.

People are infectious 1 day before
symptoms develop and 5 days after they
become sick.

Prevention:

Flu Vaccine yearly in the fall.

Pneumovax shot (one time, any time
of year),

Cover your mouth and nose when
you sneeze or cough.
  Wash your hands well and often.

HAND WASHING

1. All Personnel providing patient care are to wash their hands upon entering and leaving a residents room.
2. If gloves are worn when providing care you are to wash your hands after removing the gloves.
3. When washing your hands stay away from the sink to avoidCross contamination of your uniform.
4. Prepare your paper towel.
5. Turn on the water at a normal flow to avoid splashing.
6. Using a moderate amount of antimicrobial soap, wash hands and wrists using friction as you rub, for at least one minute.
7. Rinse your hands and wrist thoroughly under running water.
8. Dry hands completely with the paper towel you set up.
9. Using the paper towel, turn off the water.
10. Discard the paper towel in the trash can.

Chapter 8
Oxygen Therapy

Oxygen Therapy

A nasal cannula is a narrow, flexible plastic tubing used to deliver oxygen through the nostrils of patients using nasal breathing. It connects to an oxygen outlet, a tank source or compressor, on one end and has a loop at the other end with dual pronged extended openings at the top of the loop. The prongs are slightly curved to fit readily into the front portion of a patient's nostrils. The tubing of the loop is fitted over the patient's ears and is brought together under the chin by a sliding connector that holds the cannula in place.

A nasal cannula is used to deliver low concentrations of oxygen. It can deliver from 24% to 45% oxygen at a flow rate of 0.26-1.58 gal (1-6 l) per minute.

1L = 24-25%	2L = 27-29%
3L = 30-33%	4L = 33-37%
5L = 36-41%	6L = 39-45%

A simple oxygen face mask is a plastic device that is contoured to fit over a patient's nose and mouth. It is used to deliver oxygen as the patient breathes through either the nose or the mouth. A simple oxygen mask has open side ports that allow room air to enter the mask and dilute the oxygen, as well as allowing exhaled carbon dioxide to leave the containment space. It also has narrow plastic tubing fixed to the bottom of the mask that is used to connect the mask to an oxygen source. An adjustable elastic band is connected to each side of the mask and slides over the head and above the ears to hold the mask securely in place.

A simple mask is used to deliver moderate to high concentrations of oxygen. It can deliver from 40% to 60% oxygen at a flow rate of 2.64-3.17 gal (10-12 l) per minute.

A partial rebreather oxygen mask is similar to a simple face mask, however, the side ports are covered with one-way discs to prevent room air from entering the mask. This mask is called a rebreather because it has a soft plastic reservoir bag connected to the mask that conserves the first third of the patient's exhaled air while the rest escapes through the side ports. This is designed to make use of the carbon dioxide as a respiratory stimulant.

A partial rebreather mask is used to deliver high concentrations of oxygen. It can deliver 70% to 90% oxygen at a flow of 1.58-3.96 gal (6-15 l) per minute.

A non-rebreather oxygen mask is similar to a simple face mask but has multiple one-way valves in the side ports. These valves prevent room air from entering the mask but allow exhaled air to leave the mask. It has a reservoir bag like a partial rebreather mask but the reservoir bag has a one-way valve that prevents exhaled air from entering the reservoir. This allows larger concentrations of oxygen to collect in the reservoir bag for the patient to inhale.

A non-rebreather mask is used to deliver high flow oxygen. It can deliver 90% to 100% oxygen at a flow of 3.96 gal (15 l) per minute.

A Venturi oxygen mask is similar to a simple face mask but the tubing that connects to the oxygen source is larger than that of other masks. The connector has interchangeable adaptors that widen or narrow the diameter of the flow through the tubing to allow settings of specific concentrations of oxygen through the mask.

A variable flow rate mask has interchangeable adaptors that may be set to deliver oxygen at 24%, 28%, 31%, 35%, 40%, or 50%.

The use of a face mask can cause a patient to perspire and feel warm, claustrophobic or nauseated. Explain the importance of the oxygen to the patient and encourage him to relax and breathe slowly. A cold cloth on the forehead and moral support can help the patient overcome these anxious feelings. If a patient with an oxygen mask begins to vomit, quickly remove the mask. There is a danger of aspirating vomit into the lungs if it collects in the mask over the nose and mouth. Support the patient, assist them in cleaning the mouth after vomiting by rinsing with water or mouthwash, clean off the mask and the attached tubing, and replace it. The physician should be notified and antiemetics may be ordered.

Be cautious about giving oxygen to patients with chronic obstructive pulmonary disease because they may retain carbon dioxide. Oxygen may depress the hypoxic drive in these patients. They should be observed for decreased respirations, an altered mental state or further elevations of their carbon dioxide levels.

When the mask or cannula is off, the skin on the face and above the ears should be checked for signs of skin irritation. If the skin is irritated above the ears, cotton padding can be placed between the ears and the elastic band or the cannula tubing to protect the skin. If the skin of the face is irritated, the face can be massaged gently and a water-based moisturizer applied. The mask can be loosened slightly to decrease irritation. The use of petroleum ointment to the lips or nose should be avoided because it can obstruct the cannula prong openings. If a humidifier is used with the oxygen apparatus, the humidity bottle should be refilled with distilled water according to the medical setting routine or at least once every eight hours.

Complications

The most serious complication of oxygen therapy is the depression of the hypoxic drive to breathe in patients with chronic lung disease. High levels of oxygen may cause elevated levels of trapped carbon dioxide, which may lead to a decrease in respirations, a state of narcosis, and eventually to respiratory stasis or arrest.

Liquid Oxygen (LOX)

Liquid oxygen also referred to as LOX, is a versatile and efficient means of supplying oxygen to the home patient. The system usually consists of a bulk storage reservoir unit that remains in a permanent place in the home and a portable, refillable lightweight carrrying container. Both the reservoir and portable units are constructed similar to a thermos bottle consisting of an inner and outer container with a vacuum in between. Several different manufacturers produce various styles and sizes of liquid supply systems but all operate basically the same.

The bulk storage unit is normally filled with anywhere from 40 to 100 lb of liquid oxygen. However, the typical setup usually contains around 100 lb of liquid oxygen (equals 33,756 Liters of gaseous oxygen) and provides a low working pressure between 20 and 90 psig. The storage unit can be used to deliver oxygen directly to the patient or be used to refill a portable unit carried around by the patient.

The portable, refillable carrying container is filled from the storage unit when necessary. When full, the portable container weighs between 6 and 11 lbs and provides approximately 1,025 Liters of gas. The use of a permanent storage unit and a refillable portable unit allows the patient more freedom to move about.

Oxygen becomes a liquid at temperatures below its boiling point of -183°C and takes on a pale blue color weighing 1.14 times the weight of water. When the temperature of liquid oxygen is greater then -118.6°C, the liquid will return back into a gas regardless of the pressure exerted on it. This is known as the critical temperature. 1 Liter of liquid oxygen provides 860 Liters of gas.

The liquid oxygen is kept in insulated containers (called dewars). These keep the oxygen in liquid form at a temperature of -170 degrees Celius. The container consists of a lower portion where the oxygen is in a liquid state and a smaller upper portion where the liquid has evaporated creating a gas. When the unit is being used by the patient, a flow control valve is opened to deliver oxygen to the patient. This creates a pressure gradient between the gas-filled upper portion of the container (called the head pressure) and the atmospheric pressure. Liquid oxygen passes through a warming coil, is converted to a gas, and is made available for patient delivery. When the upper portion falls below a certain pressure, liquid oxygen is drawn up from the bottom of the container to provide a constant flow to the patient.

Since the cooled liquid oxygen is under pressure, the room temperature will cause some evaporation of the liquid into a gas creating more pressure in the container. This usually occurs when the container is not being used on a regular basis. When the pressure reaches a certain point a primary relief valve will open to vent to the outside. If the primary valve fails, a secondary relief valve will take over when the pressure reaches 10 psig above operating pressure. There is often a small venting of oxygen by the device as part of its normal operation.

Typical oxygen reservoirs contain approximately 40 Liters of liquid oxygen (depending on the model) that may last 8-10 days at 2-Liter/min. The controls on the portable liquid oxygen container enable the patient to select oxygen flow rates that can be used with a nasal cannula, transtracheal catheter, mask, or other oxygen delivery device. Oxygen flows are usually limited to 6 Liter/min however on most models.

Advantages of LOX

1. Comes in 30 and 40 liter capacity
2. Consumes no electricity
3. Attractive design
4. Oxygen flow rate up to 15 lpm

5. Supplies oxygen continuously for up to 11 days (at 2 lpm)

Disadvantages of LOX

1. Loud noises are made when the smaller units are filled from the larger ones.
2. The connection can become frozen if the filling is not done properly. All connections should be airtight.
3. There is evaporation loss from the cannisters when they are not in use.
4. Tank needs to be refilled regularly by a service technician.

Concentrators

Oxygen concentrators were introduced in the mid 1970s and have become a convenient, reliable source of supplemental oxygen. The air we breathe contains approximately 21% oxygen, 78% nitrogen, and 1% other gases. In a concentrator, room air passes through a regenerative adsorbent material called a molecular sieve. This material separates the oxygen from the nitrogen and other gases. The result is a constant supply of oxygen for patient use.

There are several different models and sizes of oxygen concentrators available on the market today. However, all models have the same basic parts: a power switch to turn the unit on and off, a flow selector that regulates the amount of oxygen the patient receives, an alarm system that alerts the patient if the power is interrupted and, if prescribed, a humidifier unit that allows the oxygen to be moisturized so it will not dry out to the patient's nose, mouth and throat.

The oxygen is delivered to the patient through a nasal cannula or face mask. The tubing on the cannula or mask is attached to the outlet on the humidifier unit. Sometimes, an extra length of tubing may be attached between the concentrator and the nasal cannula or face mask. This will allow the patient to move about at a farther distance from the concentrator.

It is very important that the patient use the oxygen dosage prescribed by their physician. Using too much oxygen or too little can have harmful effects.

Care of Concentrator

Cleaning and disinfecting your equipment is simple, yet very important. Proper care prevents infection. Cleaning should be done in a dust and smoke free area away from open windows.

Following are instructions for cleaning your equipment:

1. Remove the filter and wash in warm water with a non lotion detergent. Rinse thoroughly and pat dry with a clean towel.
2. Place filter back on concentrator.

Care of **Humidifier** Bottle

If you are using a humidifier bottle with your oxygen concentrator, you will need to check the water in the bottle often. **ONLY USE DISTILLED WATER IN THE HUMIDIFIER BOTTLE.** You should use your back-up oxygen whever filling or cleaning the humidifier.

Following are instructions for cleaning your

the humidifier:

1. Once a day you will need to remove the humidifier from the concentrator and discard any remaining water.
2. Rinse the bottle under tap water then refill bottle with distilled water.Screw the lid on tight making sure you do not cross thread it. **NOTE: Cross-threading the lid on the humidifier bottle will result in a loss of oxygen.**
3. Attach bottle back on the concentrator.
4. Your humidifier must be disinfected every third day using either a vinegar/water solution or a disinfectant solution that Medox Healthcare suggests. Soak for a minimum of 30 minutes then rinse and let air dry.

The patient should feel completely confident in using the home oxygen system prescribed by their physician. The patient will also be given our 24 hour number in the case of an emergency.

Page left blank

Chapter 9
Post Mortum Care

Post Mortem Care

Before you are faced with an expired resident,

Read the policies and procedures for your facility as they supersede anything you read here. Also find out the local county procedures for a coroner's case.

If you find a resident unresponsive, quickly establish their code status. If they are a full code start CPR and have someone call 911.

If they are a DNR check for a pulse peripheral and apical, check for spontaneous respirations, check for a B/P. If all of these are absent, check pupils and they will probably be fixed and not react to light. Now check the clock that is your time of death.

If they are on hospice call hospice and verify that they will contact the family, MD, and the mortuary.
Always check to see if the hospice people will be coming in. Sometimes they expect the facility to take care of these things but usually hospice takes care of everything.

If they are not on hospice, then start the calls.

If they are a coroner's case call the coroner and have the chart ready. The answering service will usually have one of the coroners call back. Be ready to site the demographics and history on the resident and they will inform you if they will be taking the body or in most cases they will give you the OK to release the body to the funeral home. Make sure you get a name of whom you spoke with.

Then place a call to the attending physician. Notify them of the time of death and be sure to get an order to release the body to the funeral home.

If you may release the body remove all the tubes (IV's, G tubes, foleys) and have the Cna's
Clean the body up and place in proper alignment. Close their eyes if they are still open.
If needed roll a towel and place under the chin to keep the mouth closed till the family gets there.
I have seen staff scramble to clean things up before rigor mortise sets in. do not rush as rigor Mortis, a stiffening of the muscles, usually starts to take place at around 3 hours after someone is dead with full rigor occurring at about 12 hours after death. After the 12 hour mark the rigor slowly ceases and at around 72 hours rigor disappears

Make sure the room looks and smells presentable.

Next call the Power of attorney, and inform them of the situation. Some nurses like to say that "the resident is not doing well" with some families when the death is expected and you can just say that they expired. Regardless of what is listed in the chart, verify what funeral home and branch they wish to use. (Some funeral homes have more than one location) Ask the family if they will be coming in, some do, some do not.

Hold off calling the funeral home till after the family either states that they are not coming in or after they leave. Some families get on the phone and call the extended family to come in, and that's fine, but they may take quite some time. If you had notified the funeral home too soon, they show up and have to wait on the family and they really do not have time for that.

 When the family leaves, you can then call the funeral home they usually want the residents name, date of birth, time of death, Power of attorney, POA's phone number and the name and phone number of the physician that will be signing the death certificate.

Your facility probably has a form for the funeral Home to sign. If they do not get a blank nurses note with the residents name on it and fill out the name, address and phone of the funeral home. Record the date and time of pick up, and list anything that was sent with. (Send wigs, dentures and eye glasses with the funeral home)
Then have the representative from the funeral home sign and record their state license number on the sheet.

Recommended documentation (Example)

6-1-09
1:18am   Resident found unresponsive, no pulse, spontaneous respirations, b/p, pupils fixed and non reactive. Time of death, 06-01-2009 01:18am.

If Required
01:20am   Bob Jones cook county coroner notified of death gave OK to release body to the funeral home.

01:22 am   Dr Ben Casey notified of death, new orders received. (then write the order, "may release body to funeral home")

01:25am   notified Mary Smith POA of death, She will be coming in.

01:50am   Family at bedside.

02:20am   Family left, Shady Rest funeral home notified, ETA, 1 hour.

03:30am   Funeral home picked up body.

Chapter 10
Tips and tricks and assorted notes

Psychotic Documentation Guide

Descriptions not to use
Agitation
Simple Pacing
Wandering
Poor Self Care
Restlesness
Crying Out (occassional)
Yelling (occassional)
Screaming (occassional)
Impaired Memory
Anxiety
Depression
Insomnia – Sleep
Unsociability
Indifference to surroundings
Fidgeting
Nervousness
Uncooperative

BEHAVIOR DESCRIPTIONS YOU CAN USE

Spitting
Bitting
Kicking
Scratching
Fighting
Slapping, Hitting, Pushing
Extreame fear
Frightful Distress
Pinching
Inappropriate sexual behavior
Pacing (Continous)
Feces finger painting
Throwing objects
Purposeful Vomiting
Tripping others
Ramming others
Head banging
Self Mutilation
Inappropriate purposeful B&B
Crying out (Continous)
Yelling (Continous)
Delusions
Paranoia
Hallucinations (Audio – visual)

Psychotropic Medications

Generic Name	Trade Name	Behavior	Aims
Alprazolam	Xanax	Anxiety	
Buspirone	Buspar	Anxiety	
Chlordiazepoxide	Librium	Anxiety	
Chlorazepate	Tranxene	Anxiety	
Diazapam	Valium	Anxiety	
Hydroxyine	Atarax, Vistaril	Anxiety	
Lorazepam	Ativan	Anxiety	
Meprobamate	Equanil	Anxiety	
Midazolam	Versed	Anxiety	
Oxazepam	Serepax	Anxiety	
Clonazepam	Klonopin	Anxiety	
Amitriptyline	Elavil	Depression	
Bupropion	Wellbutrin	Depression	
Citalopram	Celexa	Depression	
Clomipramine	Anafranil	Depression	
Desipramine	Norpramin	Depression	
Doxepin	Sinequan	Depression	
Fluoxetint	Prozac	Depression	
Imipramine	Tofranil	Depression	
Mitazapine	Remeron	Depression	
Nefazodone	Serzone	Depression	
Nortriptyline	Pamelor	Depression	
Paroxetine	Paxil	Depression	
Sertraline	Zoloft	Depression	
Escitalopram	Lexapro	Depression	
Tranylcypromine	Parnate	Depression	
Trazodone	Desyrel	Depression	

Venlafaxine	Effexor	Depression	
Generic Name	**Trade Name**	**Behavior**	**Aims**
Chloral	Nectec	Hypnotic	
Estazolam	Prosom	Hypnotic	
Flurazepam	Dalmane	Hypnotic	
Pento Barbital	Nembutal	Hypnotic	
Seco Barbital	Seconal	Hypnotic	
Temazepam	Restoril	Hypnotic	
Triazolam	Halcion	Hypnotic	
Zaleplon	Sonata	Hypnotic	
Zolpidem Tartrate	Ambien	Hypnotic	
Chlorpromazine	Thorazine	Psychotic	Y
Clozapine	Clozaril	Psychotic	Y
Fluphenazine	Prolixin	Psychotic	Y
Haloperidol	Haldol	Psychotic	Y
Loxapine	Loxitane	Psychotic	Y
Mesoridazine	Serentil	Psychotic	Y
Molindone	Moban	Psychotic	Y
Olanzapine	Zyprexa	Psychotic	Y
Perphenazine	Trlafon	Psychotic	Y
Pimozide	Orap	Psychotic	Y
Quetiapine	Seroquel	Psychotic	Y
Risperidone	Risperdal	Psychotic	Y
Thioridazine	Mellaril	Psychotic	Y
Thiothixene	Navane	Psychotic	Y
Trifluperazine	Stelazine	Psychotic	Y
Aripiprazole	Abilify	Psychotic	Y
Zyprazidone	Geodon	Psychotic	Y

Never administer a psychotropic medication till the consent is either signed or you have 2 nurse confirmation for a verbal telephone consent.

Bruising

As a person ages, he or she will bruise more easily. The layer of protective fat just under the skin becomes thinner. The small blood vessels also become more fragile and are more easily damaged. Frequent long-term exposure to the sun can also cause the skin to be more fragile and likely to bruise. A tendency to bruise easily may run in families.

There are three types of bruises:
Subcutaneous - beneath the skin.
Intramuscular - within the underlying muscle. It is often difficult to use the muscle that has been bruised.
Periosteal - bone bruise. This is the most severe and painful.
Bruises can last from days to months and usually occur in several stages. A bruise generally starts out as a pinkish-red area or as tiny red dots or blotches on the skin. The bruise may be very small and may blend in with the texture of the skin, or it may be large, swollen, and painful. Within days to a week or so, the bruise becomes more purple. As it heals, it becomes brownish-yellow. Generally,

bruises heal and disappear within 2 to 3 weeks.

Possible causes of bruising include:
Blood disorders, including problems with blood clotting such as hemophilia A or hemophilia B Blood-related diseases such as leukemia Liver disease, such as cirrhosis, Lymphomas
Certain disorders in which bone marrow cells grow at an abnormal rate.
Nutritional deficiencies, such as deficiency in vitamins C, K, B12, or folic acid, sepsis, or severe infection in the bloodstream.
Systemic lupus erythematosus (SLE)
Trauma, injury or physical abuse
Prolonged coughing or vomiting
Medications, such as blood thinners
Surgery or other medical procedures
Allergy-related disorders.

Treatment
The way one deals with bruising obviously depends on the cause. Some cases of bruising may be prevented or reduced if the cause is eliminated, such as replacing vitamins in someone who has vitamin deficiency.

Sometimes it may not be possible to determine or

treat the underlying cause. In such cases, being careful not to bang or knock the skin against hard surfaces will decrease the likelihood of developing bruises. In general, wearing protective clothing will also prevent or lessen bruising. Avoiding excessive exposure to the sun may minimize skin damage.

Some tips:
Place ice on the bruise to help it heal faster and to reduce swelling. Place the ice in a cloth, not directly on the skin. Keep the ice on the bruise for about 15 minutes per hour for the first 24-48 hours. After that, applying a hot pack to the area will help the bruise heal more quickly.
Keep the bruised area raised above the heart, if practical. This helps keep blood from pooling in the bruised tissue.
Try to rest the bruised body part by not overworking the muscles in that area.
If needed, use a pain killer such as acetaminophen (Tylenol) to help reduce the pain from the bruise.
If a person is taking a blood thinner (e.g. aspirin or warfarin), it is important that they take it exactly as prescribed in order to reduce the likelihood of bruising.

A person who has hemophilia may be given blood transfusions; a person who has nutritional deficiencies may be given special dietary recommendations; a person who has leukemia or cancer may require special medications and procedures; a person who has bacteria in the blood may need antibiotics.

Consult a doctor if...
Rarely, there will be a feeling of extreme pressure in a bruised area, especially if it is large or very painful. This may be due to a condition known as *compartment syndrome*. Increased pressure on the soft tissues and structures beneath the skin can decrease the supply of vital blood and oxygen to the tissues. This is potentially life-threatening and you should receive emergency care promptly; surgery frequently needs to be performed to relieve the extreme buildup of pressure.
You are bruising spontaneously without any injury, fall, or other cause.
There are signs of infection around the bruised area such as streaks of redness, pus or other drainage, or fever.

Healing sequence and timescale

Bruises heal over approximately 72 hours to one week. Extensive bruising will take longer. The stage of healing can be seen from the color change in the bruise:

Dark blue/purple (new) » blue » brown » green » yellow » healed

Staging of bruise age

Time	Description
0 - 2 days	Swollen and tender
0 - 5 days	Red, Purple
5 - 7 days	Green
7 - 10 days	Yellow
10 - 14 days	Brown

Survey Preparation

1. REMEMBER to knock and introduce yourself before entering a resident's room.
2. ROOM CALL CORD must be within reach of resident at all times.
3. PULL privacy curtain when performing resident care.
4. APPLY A&D Ointment AFTER EVERY CARE.
5. REMEMBER to turn and reposition residents every 2 hours.
6. CHECK residents to ensure they are properly groomed (trimmed fingernails, shaved, ect.)
7. PERFORM oral care.
8. ANSWER call lights promptly.
9. OFFER fluids often.
10. REMEMBER to wash hands before and after each resident.
11. DO NOT WEAR GLOVES in the common areas (ie, hallways, ect.)
12. REMEMBER to bag soiled linens and soiled diapers.
13. REPLACE plastic trashcan liner.
14. PLACE splints on residents NOTE: Splints are not to be worn in the dining rooms.

15. WALK TO DINE Program.
16. 02 SIGNS must be posted.
17. Beds and Bedside Care.
18. BATHROOMS-nothing on the floors. All other items left in the bathroom must be marked with resident's name. No basins or urinals on the floor in the bathroom, they must be bagged and in the nightstand bottom drawer for each resident.
19. CALL LIGHT CORDS IN BATHROOMS cannot be wrapped around grab bar.
20. USE FOLEY COVERS on Foley bags at all time. Foley bags must be opposite the door if the resident is in bed. Foley should not be hanging on the side rails.
21. PERI-WASH (big bottle of) cannot be at the bedside-PERI-SPRAY (individual) keep in bottom drawer.
22. NO extra linen or diapers in room.
23. PLASTIC TUBING from oxygen tanks and nebulizers must be in plastic bags when not in use.
24. ISOLATION- Make sure isolation cart outside with supplies and isolation sign outside on the door. Isolation set up inside the room.
25. ALL staff are mandated to wear an ID. BADGE & GATE BELT at all times

10 Reminders for med pass

1. Eye drops: wait 5 minutes between drops even if it is the same med do not give in a public area wash hands *before* and after or use gloves go in alphabetical order-drops first then gels

2.. Inhalers: wait 1 minute *before* the 2nd puff or 5 minutes before second inhaler use a spacer if possible rinse mouth after using do not use in a public area

3. Nebulizers: wash apperatus between uses nurse must stay with pt while nebulizer is running to ensure med is delivered properly and allow for privacy

4. Ear drops: resident to lie on side for 5 minutes *before* putting in the other ear

5. Do not alter a med in any way that says "DO NOT CRUSH" *If a* resident cannot swallow it-you need to get it in a liquid form or change the med.

6. You need an MD order to change from tablet to liquid

You must have an order to crush meds

7. Watch resident take their meds-don't walk away Or leave pills at the bedside

8. Sublingual: do not allow to swallow do not follow with water

9. Shaking: anything labeled suspension or has shake well label on it needs 30 seconds of shaking

10. Labeling/Expirations: YOU MUST WRITE THE DATE WHEN OPENED ON MULTI-DOSE VIALS!

11. Discard open vials after 30 days

HYDRATION

I hate sending a resident to ER only to hear that they were admitted with a diagnosis of dehydration. This implies that we were too lazy to give the resident a lousy glass of water.

I resent that.

I don't know any nurse that would refuse a resident a glass of water unless they were on a fluid restriction or were npo for some clinical reason.
This little guide will help you to track the fluid intake of at risk residents.

HYDRATION

WHO Is at risk:
Chronic diarrhea
History of Refusing Fluids
Dependence on staff for feeding
Infections process
Diuretic use
Lacking a sensation of thirst
Dysphagia
Limited fluid intake

Elevated Temperature
Renal Disease
Enteral/perenteral nutrition
Vomiting
Fecal Impaction

**WHAT...fluids are counted
and how much**

Small Juice
 Large Juice
 Milk carton
 Water glass
Coffee cup
Soup bowl
 Ice Cream
Pudding
Jell-O
Supplements

AMOUNTS
1oz = 30cc
2 oz = 60cc
3oz = 90cc
4oz = 120cc
5oz = 150cc
6oz = 180cc
7oz = 210cc
8oz = 240cc

GOAL: >1500 cc/dav

ENTERAL FEEDINGS AND MEDICATIONS

Compatibility of medications with enteral solutions:

Enteral feedings may alter the bioavailability of some medications. The most common incompatibility problems are associated with the following medications:
1quinolone antibiotics
ciprofloxacin (Cipro)
norfloxacin (Norqxin)
ofloxacin (Floxin)
levofloxacin (Levaquin)
phenytoin (Dilantin)
warfarin (Coumadin)
carbamazepine suspension
(Tegretol® suspension)
hydralazine (Apresoline)
levothyroxine (with enteral products containing soybeans)
penicillin V potassium
theophylline

It is recommended that medications in the quinolone family not be administered via a jejunostomy tube because the duodenum appears to be the predominant site for their absorption. Some medications may not be administered with enteral formulas because they form precipitates that may clog the feeding tube. The following medications are considered physically incompatible with enteral formulas:

brompheniramine/phenylephrine elixir (Dimetane®)

brompheniramine/phenylpropanolamine elixir (Dimetapp®)

calcium glubionate (Neo-Calglucon®)

chlorpromazine (Thorazine® Concentrate)

ferrous sulfate (Feosol®)

guaifenasin (Robitussin®)

lithium citrate (Cibalith-S®)

medium chain triglycende oil (MCT Oil®)

methenamine mandelate

metoclopramide l (Reglan®)

opium tincture, camphorated. elixir (Paregoric®)

potassium chloride 10% liquid, 20% liquid

pseudoephedrine (Sudafed®)

sodium biphosphate (Fleets Phospha Soda®)

sucralfate (Carafate®)

thioridazine (Mellaril® Concentrate)

zinc sulfate capsules

Understanding and dealing with resident aggression

From time to time, residents can become aggressive and, yes, violence does happen. However, these aggressive outbursts can be understood and, in many cases, prevented. In all situations the combative behavior can be managed. Staff can anticipate and in many instances de-escalate a potentially violent episode. Furthermore, once the aggressive episode is under way, there are ways in which staff can effectively intervene.

Extent of Aggressive Behavior
Although there is the cherished image of Grandma baking and handing out cookies and Grandpa fishing with the grandchildren, there is another picture of a senior citizen who is angry, shouting, kicking, and occasionally striking out at others. In fact, OSHA has found long-term care facilities to be dangerous workplaces because of resident combativeness.[1] At these facilities CNAs constitute 90% of the victims.[2] In one nursing facility, 18% of the staff noted aggression as a daily occurrence.[3] Five percent of nursing home residents will be involved with aggressive behavior each week, and 40% of nursing home aggression is

recurrent.[4] Elder aggression in the community is also significant: Elderly people with dementia residing in the community have a 65% incidence of aggressive behavior.

Causes of Aggressive Behavior

As extensive as elder aggression can be in long-term care facilities, so too can be the causes for combative behavior. When a resident lashes out it is more often than not a manifestation of an underlying condition. Just as fever can be a symptom of infection, aggression suggests the presence of a medical, psychological, or social problem.

Aggression is often the result of a medical condition. For example, a resident's outburst may reflect a urinary tract infection or pneumonia. One 76-year-old female resident would become disruptive every time she had a respiratory infection. Hence, the treatment of her aggressiveness involved the use of antibiotics. One especially important reason to look at physical causes for the aggressive behavior first is that the underlying illness may be readily treatable. Similarly, endocrine problems, medication reactions and interactions, and alcohol and drug abuse must be considered as possible causes for such behavior.

Another major contributor to aggression is dementia, defined by memory loss, disorientation, and difficulty in communication—symptoms that can lead to fear, depression, anxiety, and panic. In one study, among residents with dementia, 45% exhibited aggressive behavior within a two-week study period. Although Alzheimer's disease represents the majority of dementia cases, there are many other causes, such as head trauma, atherosclerosis, and multiple cerebral infarcts. One 66-year-old male resident with Alzheimer's would forget where he placed his glasses. When he could not find them, he would accuse staff of stealing them. Later, he would become agitated and threatening toward those around him. Things would gradually quiet down when the staff found his spectacles.

There is often a relationship between dementia and infections. When a resident with dementia contracts an infection, he may have difficulty telling others of his discomfort, and an aggressive outburst may be his way of communicating it. Based on our work in many long-term care facilities, we have found that unexpressed and unrecognized pain can lead to aggressive events.

A number of psychological problems can translate into aggressive behaviors. These include depression and a host of serious and persistent mental disorders. Depression is marked by a pervasive feeling of sadness, guilt, thoughts of death, dread, and despair, as well as physical symptoms such as a diminished appetite and difficulty with sleep. Depression is common within long-term care facilities.[6] Many people with depression also experience a sense of loss. Residents entering a long-term care facility, no matter how wonderful it may be, can experience a number of losses, including their homes and their independence. Residents also might have other losses in their lives, such as jobs, health, and loved ones. For some the contemplation of their own deaths can be depressing.[8] That depression can evolve into anger and, in turn, lead these residents to strike out at others.

For some, mental illnesses have been a persistent and lifelong struggle. These illnesses include schizophrenia, bipolar disorder (manic-depressive illness), some anxiety disorders, and post-traumatic stress disorder (PTSD). Although most of these disorders can be effectively treated with medications, sometimes a resident's symptoms emerge and can trigger an aggressive episode. For example, an 81-year-old female resident with bipolar disorder periodically would develop symptoms of mania manifested by loud singing and yelling at staff. For many residents suffering from PTSD, memories of war, the Holocaust, other incidents of genocide, or early child abuse still live in their minds and occasionally erupt into violent events.

Finally, the interpersonal social context of residents' lives can be responsible for aggressive episodes. The dynamics here can take many forms. Residents may have disagreements with their roommates or other residents. They may have conflicts with their spouses, children, or siblings. They may experience difficulties with staff. Although 85% of residents in long-term care facilities are white,[9] in many facilities staff members include people of different ethnic/racial origins. Some residents carry their lifelong prejudices into old age, and these biases may make them uncomfortable with some direct care workers.

Whatever the cause of resident aggression, each cause requires its own approach—for example, the treatment of an underlying urinary tract infection. More vexing is when several factors combine to trigger an outburst. For example, the phenomenon of "sundowning," in which residents become agitated as the sun sets, can be the result of any combination of the resident's diminished eyesight and hearing, early dementia, feelings of hunger, and disorientation caused by staff shift changes.

Prevention/De-escalation

There are 10 basic techniques for effective de-escalation. Use of these procedures can not only diminish or halt the agitation, but can improve the quality of care.

These are:
1. active listening
2. effective verbal responding
3. redirection
4. "fiblets"
5. stance
6. positioning
7. "tincture" of time
8. not jumping to conclusions
9. controlling the environment
10. Teamwork

Active listening and effective verbal responding represent the key aspects of good communication with all residents. This means taking the time to really hear what a person is saying and then thinking about the response. For example, an elderly gentleman was very upset and began angrily pacing the floor. As a CNA started to walk with him and listen to his concerns, he confided in her that his wife was late in coming to see him that day. When the CNA checked the day's schedule, she was able to reassure him in a calm, caring voice that his wife would arrive in two hours. He was relieved by this and his pacing ceased.

Residents with memory impairments benefit from the use of **redirection** and **"fiblets."** In redirection, staff simply draw the resident's attention to another subject and take her mind off of whatever she is focusing on. Fiblets are often called "little white lies." They address the subject the resident is dwelling on, provide some comfort, and allow the resident to mentally move on to another subject. In one facility, at 4 p.m. a resident became agitated because "her factory shift was up and she had to catch the bus home." She paced the floor and wanted to get on the bus. Staff recognized her daily distress, and each afternoon at 3:55 p.m. would give her a ticket for her bus and tell her to wait for it. The "ticket" was a fiblet that redirected her. After a few minutes she became interested in supper and forgot about her bus.

Attention to staff's stance and positioning in relation to an agitated resident is very important. By standing with feet about 18 inches apart, staff are able to work and move with a resident without losing their balance. Also, if they position themselves to the side rather than directly in front of a resident behaving aggressively, and maintain a distance of approximately six feet, staff are less likely to be struck by the resident—and he will feel less threatened by them, as well.

One technique of particular value is applying the **"tincture" of time**. This simply means allowing the resident to have time and space to let his/her outburst dissipate.

Not jumping to conclusions means listening to what the resident is really concerned about and then responding to it rather than assuming the obvious. For example, one day a resident began yelling. Staff assumed she was annoyed that her son had not visited that day. When her CNA asked what she was shouting about, the resident told the aide about pain she was experiencing in her right shoulder.

When a resident is becoming aggressive, there are a number of steps staff must take in **controlling the environment**. These include moving other residents and staff out of harm's way, removing objects that could be used by the resident to hurt herself or others, and blocking routes by which she could leave the facility. Staff must also make sure the agitated resident is not alone and is always kept in view.

Finally, dealing with an aggressive resident requires staff **teamwork**. The team must cooperate on many levels. When a resident is becoming agitated, several staff members working together can be very effective. It is important for each staff member to communicate with all members of the team about the resident's status. For example, if a resident has had a difficult visit from his brother in the morning, it is critical that the teams on all shifts know about the event. It is also important that direct care staff be present at treatment team meetings. They can provide firsthand observations about the resident, and they can receive medical, social, and rehabilitative information from other members of the treatment team.

A Little Humor

You cannot survive long in healthcare without a sense of humor. So here are a few thoughts.

You Know you're a nurse if...

The front of your scrubs reads.
"Nurse" Here to save your ass not kiss it

You own at least three pens that have the names of a prescription drug on them

You wash your hands BEFORE you go to the bathroom

You know there is a special place in hell for the inventor of the call light

You consider a tongue depressor an eating utensil

Eating microwave popcorn out of a clean bedpan seems totally normal

You have wondered how to set your stethoscope to stun

You can tell it is a full moon without looking at the sky

When asked, "What color is the patient's diarrhea?" you show them your shoes.

The Cat in the Hat On Aging

I cannot see
I cannot pee
I cannot chew
I cannot screw
Oh, my God, what can I do?
My memory shrinks
My hearing stinks
No sense of smell
I look like Hell
My mood is bad - - can you tell?
My body's drooping
Having trouble pooping
The Golden years have come at last
The Golden years can kiss my Ass

Common Lab Values

Test	Normal
Abg – 02	95 - 99
Abg – Base ex	-2 - -3
Abg - Hc03	21 - 28
Abg - P02	80 - 105
Abg - Pco2	35 - 45
Abg – Ph	7.35 - 7.45
Abg - Tc02	21 - 28
Cbc – Basophils	0.0 - 2.0
Cbc – Eosinophils	0.0 - 0.5
Cbc – hct	37.0 - 47.0
Cbc – Hgb	12.0 - 16.0M 11.0 - 14.0F
Cbc - Lymphocytes	0.8 - 3.0
Cbc – Mch	27.0 - 31.0
Cbc – Mcv	81.0 - 99.0
Cbc - Mean Plate Vol	7.4 - 10.4
Cbc – Monocytes	0.2 - 14.0
Cbc – Neutrophiles	1.4 - 6.8
Cbc – Platelet	150 - 450
Cbc – Rbc	4.2 - 5.4
Cbc – Rdw	11.5 - 15.5
Cbc – Wbc	4.8 - 10.8
Chm- Albumin	3.4 - 5.0
Chm- Alk Phos	42 - 141

Chm- Bun/Creat ratio	12 - 20
Chm- Calcium	8.4 - 10.2
Chm- Chloride	98 - 107
Chm- Cholesterol	140 - 220
Chm- Clucose	70 - 105
Chm- Creatinine	0.6 - 1.2
Chm- Phosphorous	2.7 - 4.5
Chm- Potassium	3.5 - 5.1
Chm- Sodium	136 - 145
Chm- Total C02	23 - 29
Chm- Totol bili	0.2 - 1.0
Chm- Triglycerides	36 - 135
Chm- Urea Nitrogen	7.0 - 18.0
Chm-Amylase	27 - 102
Chm-Lipase	7 - 60
Chm – Bun	9 - 22
Chm - C02	24 - 31
Chm – Cpk	40 - 249
Chm – Sgpt	23 - 55
Chm - Vanco P&T	P = 30 - 40 T=5 - 10
Thy - T3 uptake	0.7 - 1.3
Thy - T4	4.5 - 12.0
Thy – Tsh	0.5 - 4.7

AIC Readings

Known as hemoglobin A1C or glycosylated hemoglobin. The A1C test shows the amount of glucose that sticks to the red blood cell, which is proportional to the amount of glucose in the blood. The following A1C chart translates your percentage to provide an estimate of your average blood glucose control over the course of two to three months of diabetes management. This is based on the fact that the life cycle of red blood cells is about 120 days. So this measures the glucose that has attached to the RBCs .

A1C	Your average mean daily plasma blood sugar is around this:
%	mg/dl
12.0%	345
11.0%	310
10.0%	275
9.0%	240
8.0%	205
7.0%	170
6.0%	135
5.0%	100
4.0%	65

SIGNS AND SYMPTOMS OF CHEMICAL IMBALANCE

HYPOGLYCEMIA
(excessive insulin)
Tremors, cold/clammy skin, mental confusion, rapid/shallow respirations, fatigue, hunger, drowsiness, anxiety, headache, lack of coordination, paresthesa of tongue/mouth/lips, hallucination, hypertension, tachycardia, seizures, coma.

HYPERGLYCEMIA
(insufficient insulin)
Hot/flushed/dry skin, fruity breath odor, (polyuria), (polydipsia), (polyphagia) acute fatigue, air hunger, deep/labored respirations, mental changes, restlessness, nausea.

HYPOKALEMIA
(potassium level less than 3.5 mEq/L)
Weakness/paresthesia of extremities, muscle cramps, nausea, vomiting, diarrhea, hypoactive bowel sounds, absent bowel sounds (paralytic ileus), abdominal distention, weak/irregular pulse, postural hypotension, sob, disorientation. irritability.

HYPERKALEMIA
(potassium level greater than 5.0 mEq/L)
Diarrhea, muscle weakness, heaviness of legs, paresthesia of tongue/hands/feet, slow/ irregular pulse, decreased B/P,

abdominal cramps, oliguria, respiratory difficulty, cardiac abnormalities.

HYPONATREMIA
 (sodium level less than 130 mEq/L)
Abdominal cramping, nausea, vomiting, diarrhea, cold/clammy skin, poor skin turgor. tremors, muscle weakness, leg cramps, increased pulse rate, irritability, apprehension, hypotension, headache.

HYPERNATREMIA
(sodium level greater than 150 mEq/L)
Hot/flushed/dry skin, dry mucous membranes, fever, extreme thirst, dry/rough/red tongue, edema, restlessness, postural hypotension, ohguria.

HYPOCALCEMIA
(calcium level less than 8.4 mg/dl)
Circumoral/peripheral numbness and tingling, muscle twitching; Chvostek's sign (facial muscle spasm; test by tapping of facial nerve anterior to earlobe, just below zygomatic arch), muscle cramping, Trousseau's sign (carpopedal spasm), seizures.
arrhythmias.

HYPERCALCEMIA
(calcium level greater than 10.2 mg/dl)
Muscle hypotonicity, lack of coordination, anorexia, constipation, confusion, impaired memory, slurred speech, lethargy, acute psychotic behavior, deep bone pain, flank pain.

Controlled Substances

CLASS 1 - High abuse potential and no approved
        medical use - heroin, LSD

CLASS 2 - High abuse potential with physical
        and/or psyc depend and some medical
        use. Requires a written script
        - morphine – amphetamines

CLASS 3 - Less potential for abuse and has
        approved Uses. Telephone orders
        accepted
        .-limited codine and anabolic steroids

CLASS 4 - Low abuse potential - benzodiazapines

CLASS 5 – Medications with limited amounts of
        opiates .-antitussives and
        antidiarrheals

Calling Physicians

When calling a doctor learn from the Boy Scouts.

BE PREPARED

Skip the junk about "Oh doctor I am so sorry to bother you on a Saturday night I am sure you are trying to relax with your family and I didn't know if I should call you or not but I decieded to call you anyway"
It's his job to take call but skip to the point.

9 times out of 10 when you call a doc to say "Mary Smith has a temp of 103" and you can't think of anything clinical to say. They will answer will be.

"Send Mary to the ER for evaluation"

Now take that same call after you have done your nursing assessment, obtained vitals, and have the history and chart in hand and try it this way.

"Mary Smith has a tep of 103, and a congested cough, her right breath sounds are diminished, her O2 sats are 92% on room air. May we get a chest xray and start her on the antibiotic of your choice and as you recall she is allergic to cipro"

This doctor knows you have a plan and most of the time it will go just as you suggested. And if for some reason, Hx of chronic respiratory failure or some other reason, the doc still wants them to go out, that doc is going to hang up the phone thinking "WOW that nurse is really on top of things."

When calling labs to a doc it's good to have the lab value but also have prior labs to report a trend. Know what meds and doses they are on.

Especially for a PT/INR know the previos INR Know what dose of coumidin they are on, when was the last change. In short

BE PREPARED

This page blank

Things I have learned about Nursing that were not taught in Nursing school

Things I learned in Kindergarten
Play fair.

Put things back where you found them.

Clean up your own mess.

Don't take things that aren't yours.

Say you're sorry when you hurt somebody.

Wash your hands before you eat. .

Live a balanced life.

Be aware of wonder.

Things that I learned from my Dog

When it's in your interest, practice obedience.

Avoid biting, when a simple growl will do.

No matter how often you're scolded, don't buy into the guilt thing and pout

If what you want lies buried, dig until you find it.

When someone is having a bad day, be silent, sit close by

Things that I have learned from Star Wars

Be careful of your overconfidence, it may really be your weakness

Try not. Do or do not…. There is no try.

Mind what you have learned, save you it can."

Be prepared for things to go wrong.

Don't give into your anger.

If you do not believe, you will always fail

Your insight serves you well.

You can't escape your destiny

Pass on what you have learned you must

Things I Learned Drinking Coffee

I am productive! I am productive! I am productive!

We all have to do the daily grind.

Automatic drip defines many people's
personalities.

Stand your grounds. .

There's no rest for the caffeinated.

There is no such thing as a free refill.

Things I Learned From Computers

Don't byte off more than you can process. .

Some people just can't hack it.

You can never tell when you're going to crash. .

If you've got a lot of Internal Drive, you'll
probably go far.

Some times it's just impossible to get Booted Up.

It's okay if you need a little tech support now and
then.

Things I learned from Santa

Encourage people to believe in you.

Always remember who's naughty and who's nice.

Don't pout.

Make your presents known.

Things I Learned From Noah's Ark

Plan ahead. It wasn't raining when Noah built the ark.

Don't listen to gossip. Do what has to be done.

For safety's sake, travel in pairs.

Don't forget that we're all in the same boat.

Remember that the woodpeckers INSIDE are often a bigger threat than the storm outside.

No matter how bleak it looks, there's always a rainbow on the other side.

DON'T MISS THE BOAT !!!!

Things I Learned From the Easter Bunny

Don't put all your eggs in one basket.

Everyone needs a friend who is all ears.

Don't count your chickens before they are hatched.

There's no such thing as too much candy.

All work and no play can make you a basket case.

Let happy thoughts multiply like rabbits.

Keep your paws off other people's jellybeans.

The grass is always greener in someone else's basket.

To show your true colors you have to come out of your shell.

Things I Learned From Trees

It's important to have roots.

In today's complex world, it pays to branch out.

If you really believe in something, don't be afraid to go out on a limb.

Be flexible so you don't break when a harsh wind blows.

Sometimes you have to shed your old bark in order to grow.

It's perfectly okay to be a late bloomer.

Avoid people who would like to cut you down.

You can't hide your true colors as you approach your autumn

It's more important to be honest than poplar.

Things That I Have Learned From My Patients

I'm not as smart as I thought I was

You can't make someone do something they don't
want to do

Stress is not for staff only

Family comes first

Where there is a will, there is a relative

Live for today

Being able to speak several languages is nice,

Knowing when to be quiet in all of them is crucial.

There are not enough words in the English
language that can equal a warm smile

I can learn to accept watching someone die

I can never accept watching someone,

who is watching someone they love, die.

No matter how much I care, some people just don't
care back.

You can get by on charm for about 15 minutes,
after that you better know something.

No matter how thin you slice it, there are always two sides.

It's taking me a long time to become the person I want to be.

It's a lot easier to react than to think things thru.

You should always leave loved ones with loving words for it may be the last time you see them.

We are responsible for what we do no matter what our mood is.

Not forgiving others becomes your baggage not theirs.

People will not always remember exactly what you said, or exactly what you did. But they will NEVER forget how you made them feel.

Abbreviations

	Abbreviation	Medical Term
A	AAA	Abdominal Aortic Aneurysm
	AAD	Antibiotic-associated diarrhea
	AAO	Alert, awake and oriented
	AAS	Acute Abdominal Series
	AB	Abortion
	ab, abs	Abdomen or Abdominal
	ABD	Abdomen
	ABE	Acute Bacterial Endocarditis
	ABG	Arterial Blood Gas
	ABI	Acquired Brain Injury
	AC	Before eating
	ACB	Aortocoronary Bypass
	ACD	Anemia of Chronic Disease
	ACE	Angiotensin-Converting Enzyme
	ACL	Anterior Cruciate Ligament
	ACLS	Advanced Cardiac Life Support
	ACS	Acute Coronary Syndrome
	ACTH	Adrenocorticotropic Hormone
	AD	Alzheimer's Disease
	ADA	Adenosine Deaminase
	ADD	Attention Deficit Disorder
	ADH	Antidiuretic Hormone
	ADHD	Attention Deficit Hyperactivity Disorder
	ADR	Adverse Drug Reaction

ADR	Acute Dystonic Reaction
AE	Hyperkalemia
AED	Antiepileptic Drug
AED	Automated External Defibrillator
AF	Atrial Fibrillation or afebrile
AF	Amniotic Fluid
AFB	Acid Fast Bacteria
AFP	Alpha-fetoprotein
AGN	Acute Glomerulonephritis
AI	Artificial Insemination or Aortic Insufficiency
AIDS	Acquired Immune Deficiency Syndrome
AIDP	Acute Infectious and Parasitical Diseases
AIDP	Autoimmune Progesterone Dermatitis
AIDP	Acute Inflammatory Demyelinating Polyneuropathy
AIN	Acute Interstitial Nephritis
AKA	Above the Knee Amputation
ALA	Aminolevulinic Acid
Alc	Alcohol
ALD	Alcoholic Liver Disease
ALG	Antilymphocytic Globulin
ALI	Acute Lung Injury
ALL	Acute Lymphoblastic Leukemia
ALP	Alkaline Phosphatase

ALPS	Autoimmune Lymphoproliferative Syndrome
ALS	Amyotrophic Lateral Sclerosis
ALT	Alanine Transaminase
amb	Ambulate
AMI	Acute Myocardial Infarction
AML	Acute Myeloid Leukemia
AMS	Acute Mountain Sickness
ANA	Anti-nuclear Antibody
ANS	Autonomic Nervous System
AODM	Adult-Onset Diabetes Mellitus (Type 2 Diabetes)
AOM	Acute Otitis Media
APC	Atrial Premature Contraction
APD	Adult Polycystic Disease
APECED	Autoimmune Polyendocrinopathy-Candidiasis-ectodermal dystrophy
APH	Antepartum Hemorrhage
APKD	Adult Polycystic Kidney Disease
APLS	Antiphospholipid Syndrome
APR	Abdominoperineal Resection
APS	Autoimmune Polyendocrine/Polyglandular Syndrome
APTT	Activated Partial

	Thromboplastin Time
ARC	AIDS-related Complex
ARDS	Acute Respiratory Distress Syndrome
ARF	Acute Renal Failure
Arg	Arginine
ARM	Artificial Rupture of Membranes
ART	Antiretroviral Therapy
ARVC	Arrhythmogenic Right Ventricular Cardiomyopathy
ARVD	Arrhythmogenic Right Ventricular Dysplasia
AS	Aortic Stenosis
ASA	Acetylsalicylic Acid (Aspirin)
ASAP	As soon as possible
ASCAD	Arteriosclerotic Coronary Artery Disease
ASCVD	Arteriosclerotic Vascular Disease (Arteriosclerosis)
ASD	Autism Spectrum Disorder
ASD	Atrial Septal Defect
ASGUS	Atypical Squamous Glandular Cells of Undetermined Significance
ASH, ASHD	Arteriosclerotic Heart Disease (Coronary Heart Disease)
ASIS	Anterior Superior Iliac Spine
ASO	Antistreptolysin-O

	AST	Aspartate Transaminase
	ATN	Acute Tubular Necrosis
	ATNR	Asymmetrical Tonic Neck Reflex
	ATP	Adenosine triphosphate
	ATP	Acute Thrombocytopenic Purpura
	ATS	Anti-tetanus Serum
	AV	Arteriovenous/Atrioventricular
	AVM	Arteriovenous Malformation
	AVR	Aortic Valve Replacement
	AXR	Abdominal X-Ray
	AZT	Azidothymidine
	a.a.	Amino Acids
	A-a gradient	Alveolar to Arterial Gradient
	A/G	Albumin/Globulin ratio
	A-V	Arteriovenous
	A-VO2	Arteriovenous Oxygen
B	BAC	Blood Alcohol Content
	BAL	Blood Alcohol Level
	BAL	Bronchoalveolar Lavage
	BAO	Basic Acid Output
	BAT	Brown Adipose Tissue
	BBB	Bundle Branch Block
	BBB L	Left Bundle Branch Block
	BBB R	Right Bundle Branch Block
	BC	Blood Culture

BCAA	Brached Chain Amino Acid
BCC	Basal Cell Carcinoma
BCG	Bacille Calmette-Guerin (Tuberculosis Vaccination)
BCP	Birth Control Pill
BD	Bipolar Disorder
BDD	Body Dysmorphic Disorder
BDI	Beck Depression Inventory
BE	Barium Enema
BEE	Basal Energy Expenditure
BGAT	Blood Glucose Awareness Training
BGL	Blood Glucose Level
bid	Twice a day
BiPAP	Bilevel Positive Airway Pressure
BiVAD	Bilateral Ventricular Assist Device
BK	Bradykinin
BKA	below-the-knee amputation
bld	Blood
BM	Bone Marrow
BM	Bowel Movement
BMC	Bone Mineral Content
BMD	Bone Mineral Density
BMI	Body Mass Index
BMP	Blood Metabolic Profile
BMR	Basal Metabolic Rate

BMT	Bone Marrow Transplant
BNP	Brain Natriuretic Peptide
BOM	Bilateral Otitis Media
BOOP	Bronchiolitis Obliterans Organizing Pneumonia
BP	Blood Pressure
BPAD	Bipolar Affective Disorder
BPD	Borderline Personality Disorder
BPH	Benign Prostatic Hyperplasia
BPM	Beats Per Minute
BPPV	Benign Paroxysmal Positional Vertigo
BRBPR	Bright Red Blood Per Rectum
BRCA 1	Breast Cancer 1 (human gene and protein)
BS	Blood Sugar
BS	Breathe Sound, Bowel Sounds
BSA	Body Surface Area
BSE	Bovine Spongiform Encephalopathy
BSL	Blood Sugar Level
BRBPR	Bright Red Blood Per Rectum
BRP	Bathroom Priviledges
BT	Bleeding Time
BTL	Bilateral Tubal Ligation
BTP	Breakthrough pain
BUN	Blood Urea Nitrogen

	BVP	Biventricular Vaginosis
	BW	Body Weight
	BX	Biopsy
C	CA	Carcinoma
	CA	Cancer
	Ca	Calcium
	CAA	Crystalline Amino Acids
	CABG	Coronary Artery Bypass Graft Surgery
	CAD	Coronary Artery Disease
	CADASIL	Cerebral Autosomal Dominant Arteriopathy with Subcortical Infarcts and Leukoencephalopathy
	CAG	Coronary Artery Graft
	CAG	Coronary Angiography
	CAH	Chronic Active Hepatitis
	CAH	Congenital Adrenal Hyperplasia
	cAMP	Cyclic Adenosine Monophosphate
	CAPD	Central Auditory Processing Disorder
	CAPD	Continuous Ambulatory Peritoneal Dialysis
	Caps	Capsule
	CAT	Computed Axial Tomography
	CBC	Complete Blood Count
	CBG	Capillary Blood Gas

CBS	Chronic Brain Syndrome
cc	Cardiac Catheter
CC	Chief Complaint
CCF	Congestive Cardiac Failure
CCK	Cholecystokinin
CCR	Cardiocerebral Resuscitation
CCU	Coronary Care Unit
CCU	Clean Catch Urine
CCV	Critical Closing Volume
CDH	Congenital Dislocated Hip
CDP	Cytosine Diphosphate
CEA	Carcinoembryonic Antigen, Carotid Endarterectomy
CF	Cystic Fibrosis
CFS	Chronic Fatigue Syndrome
CGL	Chronic Granulocytic Leukemia
cGMP	Cyclic Guanosine Monophosphate
CGN	Chronic Glomerulonephritis
CH	Congenital Hypothyroidism
CHD	Chronic Heart Disease
CHD	Coronary Heart Disease
ChE	Cholinesterase
CHF	Congestive Heart Failure
CHO	Carbohydrate
Chol	Cholesterol
CHT	Congenital Hypothyroidism

CI	Cardiac Index
CICU	Cardiac Intensive Care Unit
CIDP	Chronic Inflammatory Demyelinating Polyneuropathy
Circ	Circumcision
CIS	Carcinoma in situ
CJD	Creutzfeldt-Jakob Disease
CKD	Chronic Kidney Disease
CKMB	MB isoenzyme of creatine kinase
CLL	Chronic Lymphocytic Leukemia
CML	Chronic Myelogenous Leukemia/Chronic Myeloid Leukemia
CMML	Chronic Myelomonocytic Leukemia
CMP	Cytosine Monophosphate
CMS	Chronic Mountain Sickness
CMV	Cyomegalovirus
CN	Cranial Nerves
CNS	Central Nervous System
CO	Cardiac Output, Carbon Monoxide
CO2	Carbon Dioxide
COAD	Chronic Obstructive Airways Disease
COCP	Combined Oral Contraceptive Pill

COLD	Chronic Obstructive Lung Disease
Conj	Conjunctiva
COPD	Chronic Obstructive Pulmonary Disease
COX-1	Cyclooxygenase 1
CP	Cerebral Palsy
CP	Chest Pain
CPAP	Continuous Positive Airway Pressure
CPK	Creatine Phosphokinase
CPKMB	Creatine Phosphokinase heart
CPP	Cerebral Perfusion Pressure
CPR	Cardiopulmonary Resuscitation
CPT	Current Procedural Terminology
CrCl	Creatinine Clearance
CREST	Calcinosis Raynaud Esophagus Sclerosis Teleangiectasiae
CRF	Chronic Renal Failure
CRF	Corticotropin-releasing factor
CRH	Corticotropin-releasing hormone
CRI	Chronic Renal Insufficiency
CRNS	Certified Registered Nurse Anesthetist
CRP	C-Reactive Protein
CRT	Cardiac Resynchronization Therapy
CsA	Ciclosporin A

CSF	Cerebrospinal Fluid
CT	Computerized Tomography
CTA	Computed Tomography Angiography
CTP	Cytosine Triphosphate
CTS	Carpal Tunnel Syndrome
CTU	Cancer Treatment Unit
CTX	Ceftriaxone Contractions
CV	Cardiovascular
CVA	Costovertebral Angle
CVA	Cerebrovascular Accident
CVAT	CVA tenderness
CVC	Central Venous Catheter
CVC	Chronic Venous Congestion
CVD	Cardiovascular Disease
CVI	Cardiovascular incident
CVID	Common Variable Immunodeficiency
CVP	Central Venous Pressure
CVS	Cardiovascular System
CXR	Chest X-Ray
C/O	Complaining of
C&S	Culture & Sensitivity
C-Section	Cesarean Section
D	D5W	5% dextrose in water
	DAT	Direct Antiglobulin Test
	DAT	Diet as tolerated

DAW	Dispense as written
DBP	Diastolic Blood Pressure
DBS	Deep Brain Stimulation
DBT	Dialectical Behavioral Therapy
DC	Discharge or Discontinue
DCBE	Double Contrast Barium Enema
DCIS	Ductal Carcinoma in situ
DCM	Dilated Cardiomyopathy
DDD	Daily Defined Doses
DDS	Doctor of Dental Surgery
DDx	Differential Diagnosis
DES	Diethylstilbestrol
Detox	Detoxification
DEXA	Dual Energy X-ray Absorptionmetry
DHE	Dihydroergotamine
DHEA	Dehydroepiandrosterone
DHEA-S	Dehydroepiandrosterone Sulphate
DHF	Decompensated Heart Failure
DI	Diabetes Insipidus
DIC	Disseminated Intravascular Coagulation
DID	Dissociative Identity Disorder
DIP	Distal Interphalangeal Joint
DiPer Te	Diphtheria Pertussis Tetanus
Dis	Dislocation

DiTe	Diphtheria Tetanus
DIU	Death in Utero-Stillbirth
DJD	Degenerative Joint Disease (Osteoarthritis)
DKA	Diabetic Ketoacidosis
dl	Deciliter
DLE	Disseminated Lupus Erythematosus
DM	Diabetes Mellitus
DMD	Duchenne Muscular Dystrophy
DMD	Doctor of Dental Medicine
DNA	Deoxyribonucleic acid
DNR	Do not resuscitate
DO	Doctor of Osteopathy
DOA	Drugs of Abuse
DOA	Dead on Arrival
DOB	Date of Birth
DOE	Dyspnea on Exertion
DP	Dorsalis Pedis
DPH	Diphenylhydantoin
DPL	Diagnostic Peritoneal Lavage
DPT	Diphtheria Pertussis Tetanus-DPT vaccine
DSA	Digital Subtraction Angiography
DSM	Diagnostic and Statistical Manual
DT	Diphtheria Tetanus

	DT	Delirium Tremens
	DTA	Descending Thoracic Aorta
	DTP	Diphtheria Tetanus Pertussis
	DTR	Deep Tendon Reflex
	DU	Duodenal Ulcer
	DUB	Dysfunctional Uterine Bleeding
	DVT	Deep Vein Thrombosis
	DX	Diagnosis
	dz	Disease
	D & C	Dilation and curettage
	D/C	Discharge
	d.d.	Differential Diagnosis
E	EAA	Essential Amino Acids
	EACA	Epsilon-aminocaproic acid
	EBL	Estimated blood loss
	EBM	Expressed Breast Milk
	EBT	Electron beam tomography
	EBV	Epstein-Barr Virus
	ECF	Extracellular fluid
	ECG	Electrocardiogram
	ECHO	Echocardiogram
	ECMO	Extracorporeal Membrane Oxygenation
	ECT	Electroconvulsive Therapy
	ED	Erectile Dysfunction
	ED	Ectodermal Dysplasia
	EDD	Estimated Date of Delivery

EDH	Epidural Hematoma
EDM	Esophageal Doppler Monitor
EDTA	Ethylene-diamine-tetra-acetic acid
EEG	Electroencephalogram
EEX	Electrodiagnosis
EF	Ejection Fraction
EFAD	Essential Fatty Acid Deficiency
EGD	Esophagogastroduodenoscopy
EI	Emotional Intelligence
EKG	Electrocardiogram
ELISA	Enzyme-linked Immunosorbent Assay
EmBx	Endometrial Biopsy
EMF	Endomyocardial Fibrosis
EMG	Electromyography
EMR	Electronic Medical Record
EMU	Early Morning Urine Sample
EMV	Eyes, motor, verbal response
ENT	Ear, Nose and Throat
EOM	extraocular Muscles
EOMI	Extraocular Movements Intact
EPH	Edema Proteinuria Hypertension
EPO	Erythropoietin
EPS	Electrophysiology
EQ	Emotional Intelligence Quotient
ER	Emergency Room

	ERCP	Endoscopic Retrograde Cholangiopancreatography
	ESBL	Extended Spectrum Beta-Lactamase
	ESR	Erythrocyte Sedimentation Rate
	ESRD	End-Stage Renal Disease
	ESV	End-systolic Volume
	ESWL	Extracorporeal Shock Wave Lithotripsy
	ET	Endotracheal
	Etiol	Etiology
	ETOH	Ethanol
	ETS	Endoscopic Thoracic Sympathectomy
	ETT	Endotracheal Tube
	EUA	Examination under Anesthesia
	EUP	Extrauterine Pregnancy
	EUS	Endoscopic Ultrasonography
	EVAR	Endovascular Aneurysm Repair
	EVF	Erythrocyte Volume Fraction
	Exam	Examination
	Exp Lap	Exploratory Laparotomy
	E. Coli	Escherichia Coli bacteria
F	F	Fahrenheit
	Fab	Fragment Antigen Binding
	FAMMM	Familial Atypical Multiple Mole Melanoma Syndrome
	FAP	Familial Adenomatous Polyposis

FB	Foreign Body
FBC	Full Blood Count
FBE	Full Blood Exam
FBG	Fasting Blood Glucose
FBS	Fasting Blood Sugar
FDA	Food and Drug Administration
FDC	Follicular Dendritic Cells
FDIU	Foetal Demise in Utero
FDP	Fibrin Degradation Product
Fe	Iron
fem	Female
FEV	Forced Expiratory Volume
FFA	Free Fatty Acids
FFP	Fresh Frozen Plasma
FHR	Fetal Heart Rate
FHS	Fetal Heart Sound
FHT	Fetal Heart Tones
FHx	Family History
Flu	Influenza
FMF	Fetal Movements Felt
FMP	First Menstruation Period (Menarche)
fMRI	Functional Magnetic Resonance Imaging
FNA	Fine Needle Aspiration
FNAB	Fine Needle Aspiration Biopsy
FNAC	Fine Needle Aspiration Cytology

	FNC	Full Nursing Care
	FNH	Focal Nodular Hyperplasia
	FOBT	Fecal Occult Blood Test
	FOS	Full of Stool
	FPG	Fasting Plasma Glucose
	FRC	Functional Residual Capacity
	FROM	Full Range of Motion
	FSBS	Finger-stick Blood Sugar
	FSE	Fetal Scalp Electrode
	FSH	Follicle-stimulating Hormone
	FTA	Fluorescent Treponemal Antibody
	FTA-ABS	Fluorescent Treponemal Antibody Absorption
	FTT	Failure to thrive
	FU	Follow-up
	FUO	Fever of Unknown Origin
	FVC	Forced Vital Capacity
	FWB	Full Weight Bearing
	Fx, #	Fracture
	F/C	Fevers and/or Chills
G	G	Gravidity
	G6PD	Glucose-6-Phosphate Dehydrogenase
	GA	General Anaesthesia
	GABA	Gamma-Aminobutyric Acid
	GAD	Generalized Anxiety Disorder

GB	Gallbladder
GBM	Glomerular Basement Membrane
GC	Gonorrhea or Gonococcus
GCA	Giant Cell Arteritis
GCS	Glasgow Coma Scale
GDA	Gastroduodenal Artery
GDLH	Glutamate Dehydrogenase
GDP	Guanosine Diphosphate
GERD	Gastroesophageal Reflux Disease
GETT	General by Endotracheal Tube
GFR	Glomerular Filtration Rate
GGT	Gamma Glutamyl Transpeptidase
GH	Growth Hormone
GHFR	Growth Hormone Releasing factor
GI	Glycemic Index
GI	Gastrointestinal
GIFT	Gamete Intrafallopian Transfer
GIST	Gastrointestinal Stromal Tumor
GIT	Gastrointestinal Tract
GITS	Gastrointestinal Therapeutic System
GMC	General Medical Condition
GMP	Guanosine Monophosphate
GM-CSF	Granulocyte-Monocyte-Colony

		Stimulating Factor
	GN	Glomerulonephritis (Nephritis)
	GnRH	Gonadotropin-Releasing Hormone
	GOAT	Galveston Orientation and Amnesia Test
	GOD	Glucose Oxidase
	Gomer	Get Outta My ER
	GORD	Gastroesophageal Reflux Disease
	GOT	Glutamic-oxalacetic Transaminase
	GPT	Glutamic-pyruvic transaminase
	gr	Grain
	GRAV I	First Pregnancy
	GSW	Gun Shot Wound
	GTT	Glucose Tolerance Test
	GU	Gastric Ulcer
	GU	Genitourinary
	GVHD	Graft-versus-host disease
	Gym	Gymnasium
	Gyn	Gynecology
	GXT	Graded Exercise Tolerance (stress test)
H	HA, H/A	Headache
	HA	Hypertonia Arterialis
	HAA	Hepatitis Associated Antigen
	HAART	Highly Active Anti-aetroviral

171

	Therapy
HACE	High Altitude Cerebral Edema
HAD	HIV-associated dementia
HAE	Hereditary Angioedema
HAPE	High Altitude Pulmonary Edema
HAV	Hepatitis A Virus
Hb	Hemoglobin
HB	Heart Block
HbA	Hemoglobin A
HbA1C	Glycosylated hemoglobin
HbF	Fetal Hemoglobin
HBP	High Blood Pressure
HBsAg	Hepatitis B Surface Antigen
HBV	Hepatitis B Virus
HCC	Hepatocellular Carcinoma
hCG	Human Chorionic Gonadotropin
HCL	Hairy Cell Leukemia
Hct	Hematocrit
HCT	Hematopoietic Cell Transplantation
HCTZ	Hydrochlorothiazide
HCV	Hepatitis C Virus
HD	Hodgkin's Disease
HDL	High-density lipoprotein
HDL-C	High-density lipoprotein-cholesterol
HDU	High Dependancy Unit

HDV	Hepatitis D virus
HEENT	Head, Eyes, Ears, Nose, Throat
HELP, HELLP	Hypertension, Elevated Liver enzymes, Low Platelets
HEMA	Hydroxy Ethyl Methacrylate
Hema	Hematest
HES	Hydroxyethyl Starch
HETE	Hydroxyeicosatetraenoic Acid
HEV	Hepatitis E Virus
Hgb	Hemoglobin
HGH	Human Growth Hormone
HGPRTase	Hypoxanthine-guanine Phosphoribosyl Transferase
HGV	Hepatitis G Virus
HH	Hiatus Hernia
HHT	Hereditary Hemorrhagic Telangiectisia
HHV	Human Herpesvirus
HI	Homicidal Ideation
Hib	Haemophilus Influenzae B
HIDS	Hyper-IgD Syndrome
HIT	Heparin-induced Thrombocytopenia
HIV	Human Immunodeficiency Virus
HJR	Hepatojugular Reflex
HL	Hepatic Lipase
HL	Hodgkin's Lymphoma

HL	Hearing Level
HLA	Human Leukocyte Antigen
HLA	Histocompatibility Locus Antigen
HLHS	Hypoplastic Left Heart Syndrome
HMD	Hyaline Membrane Disease
HMGR	3-hydroxy-30methyl-glutaryl-CoA reductase
HMG-CoA	3-hydroxy-3-methyl-glutaryl-CoA
HMS	Hyper-reactive Malarial Splenomegaly
HMSN	Hereditary Motor Sensory Neuropathy
HN	Hemagglutinin-neuraminidase
HND	Hemolytic Disease of the Newborn
HNPCC	Hereditary Nonpolyposis Colorectal Cancer
HOB	Head of Bed
HOCM	Hypertrophic Obstructive Cardiomyopathy
HONK	Hyperosmolar Nonketotic Coma
HPA	Hypothalamic-Pituiatary-Adrenal Axis
HPETE	Hydroxyeicosatetraenoic Acid
HPF	High Power Field (Microscopy)

HPI	History of Present Illness
HPOA	Hypertrophic Pulmonary Osteoarthropathy
HPL	Human Placental Lactogen
HPV	Human Papillomavirus
HR	Heart Rate
HRT	Hormone Replacement Therapy
hs	Hours of Sleep
HSC	Human Chorionic Somatomammotropin
HSG	Hysterosalpingogram
HSM	Hepatosplenomegaly
HSP	Henoch-Schonlein Purpura
HSV	Herpes Simplex Virus
HT, HTN	Hypertension
Ht	Height
HTLV	Human T-lymphotropic Virus
HTPA	Hypothalamic-pitutary-adrenal axis
HTVD	Hypertensive Vascular Disease
HUS	Hemolytic Uremic Syndrome
HVLT	High-velocity Lead Therapy
Hx	History (medical)
h/o	History of
H/H	Henderson-Hasselbach Equation
H & E	Hematoxylin and Eosin
H & H	Hemoglobin and Hematocrit

	h.s.	At Bedtime
	H-S	Heel-to-shin test
	H&M	Hematemesis and Melena
	H&P	History and Physical Examination
I	I131	Radioactive Iodine
	IA	Intra-arterial
	IABP	Intra-aortic Balloon Pump
	IAI	Intra-amniotic Infection
	IBC	Inflammatory Breast Cancer
	IBD	Inflammatory Bowel Disease
	IBS	Irritable Bowel Syndrome
	IC	Informed Consent
	IC	Intensive Care
	IC	Ileocecal
	IC	Immunocompromised
	IC	Interstitial Cystitis
	IC	Immune Complex
	IC	Intracardiac
	ICCU	Intensive Cardiac Care Unit
	ICD	Implantable Cardioverter-defibrillator
	ICDS	Integrated Child Development Services Program
	ICD-10	International Classification of Diseases - 10th revision
	ICF	Intracellular Fluid

ICG	Impedance Cardiography
ICH	Intracerebral Hemorrhage
ICP	Intracranial Pressure
ICS	Intercostal Space
ICU	Intensive Care Unit
ID	Infectious Disease or Identifying Data or Identification
IDA	Iron Deficiency Anemia
IDC	Idiopathic Dilated Cardiomyopathy
IDC	Indwelling Catheter
IDC	Infiltrating Ductal Carcinoma
IDDM	Insulin Dependent Diabetes Mellitus
IDL	Intermediate Density Lipoprotein
IDP	Infectious Disease Precautions/Process
IF	Immunofluorescence
IFG	Impaired Fasting Glycaemia
Ig	Immunoglobulin
IgA	Immunoglobulin A
IgD	Immunoglobulin D
IgE	Immunoglobulin E
IgG	Immunoglobulin G
IgM	Immunoglobulin M
IGT	Impaired Glucose Tolerance
IHC	Immunohistochemistry

IHD	Ischemic Heart Disease
IHSS	Idiopathic Hypertropic Subaortic Stenosis
IM	Intramuscular
IMA	Inferior Mesenteric Artery
IMB	InterMenstrual Bleed
IMI	Intramuscular Injection
IMN	Infectious Mononucleosis
IMS	Irritable Male Syndrome
IMT	Intima-media Thickness
IMV	Intermittent Mandatory Ventilation
Inc	Incomplete
Inf	Injection
INF	Intravenous Nutritional Fluid
INH	Isoniazid
IO	Intraosseous Infusion
IOL	Induction Of Labor
IOP	Intraocular Pressure
IP	Interphalangeal Joint
IPPB	Intermittent Positive Pressure Breathing
IPPV	Intermittent Positive Pressure Ventilation
IPS	Intra-Peritoneal Sounds
IQ	Intelligence Quotient
IRDM	Insulin Resistant Diabetes Mellitus

ISA	Intrinsic Sympathomimetic Activity
ISDN	Isosorbide dinitrate
ISH	Isolated Systolic Hypertension
ISMN	Isosorbide Mononitrate
IT	Interthecal
ITP	Idiopathic Thrombocytopenic Purpura
ITU	Intensive Treatment/Therapy Unit
IU	International Units
IUCD	Intrauterine Contraceptive Device
IUD	Intrauterine Death
IUD	Intrauterine Device
IUFD	Intrauterine Foetal Demise
IUI	Intrauterine Insemination
IUP	Intrauterine Pregnancy
IUS	Intrauterine System
IV	Intravenous
IVC	Intravenous Cholangiogram
IVC	Inferior Vena Cava
IVDU	Intravenous Drug User
IVF	In vitro fertilization
IVF	Intravenous Fluids
IVP	Intravenous Pyelogram
IVPB	Intravenous Piggyback

	IVU	Intravenous Urogram
	IVUS	Intravascular Ultrasound
	IV-DSA	Intravenous Digital Subtraction Angiography
	I&D	Incision and Drainage
	I&O	Inputs and Outputs, Intake and Outputs
	i.s.q.	No change
J	JIA	Juvenile Idiopathic Arthritis
	JMS	Junior Medical Student
	JODM	Juvenile-Onset Diabetes Mellitus
	JRA	Juvenile Rheumatoid Arthritis
	JVD	Jugular Vein Distension
	JVP	Jugular Venous Pressure
K	K	Potassium
	KA	Ketoacidosis
	KBr	Potassium Bromide
	Kcal	Kilocalorie
	KCCT	Kaolin Cephalin Clotting Time
	kg	Kilogram
	KIV	Keep in View
	KLS	Kidney, Liver, Spleen
	KOR	Keep Open Rate
	KS	Kaposi's Sarcoma
	KSHV	Kaposi's sarcoma-associated Herpes virus
	KUB	Kidneys, Ureters and Bladder

	KVO	Keep Vein Open
L	L	Leukocytes (White Blood Cells)
	L	Lumbar vertebrae
	LA	Left Atrium, Lymphadenopathy
	Lab	Laboratory
	LABBB	Left Anterior Bundle Branch Block
	LAD	Left Anterior Descending-Coronary Artery
	LAD	Leukocyte Adhesion Deficiency
	LAD	Left Axis Deviation-Electrocardiogram
	LAD	Lymphadenopathy
	LAE	Left Atrial Enlargement
	LAHB	Left Anterior Hemiblock
	Lam	Laminectomy
	LAP	Leukocyte Alkaline Phosphatase
	Lap	Laparotomy
	LAR	Low Anterior Resection
	LARP	Left-Anterior, Right-Posterior
	LAS	Lymphadenopathy Syndrome
	LASIK	Laser-Assisted In-Situ Keratomileusis
	Lat	Lateral
	lb, LB	Pound
	LBBB	Left Bundle Branch Block
	LBO	Large Bowel Obstruction

LBP	Low Back Pain
LCA	Left Coronary Artery
LCIS	Lobular Carcinoma in situ
LCM	Lymphocytic Meningitis
LCX	Left Circumflex Artery
Lc of ch	Laxative of choice
LDH	Lactate Dehydrogenase
LDL	Low Density Lipoprotein
LDL-C	Low Density Lipoprotein Cholesterol
LE	Lupus Erythematosus
LE	Lower Extremity
LEC	Lupus Erythematosus Cell
LES	Lower Esophageal Sphincter
LES	Lupus Erythematosus Systemicus
leu	Leukocytes
LFT	Liver Function Test
LGL	Lown-Ganong-Levine Syndrome
LGM	Lymphogranulomatosis Maligna
LGV	Lymphogranuloma Venereum
LH	Luteinizing Hormone
Lig	Ligament
LIH	Left Inguinal Hernia
LLE	Left Lower Extremity
LLL	Left Lower Lobe
LLQ	Left Lower Quadrant

LM	Left Main
LMA	Left Mentoanterior-Fetal Position
LMCA	Left Main Coronary Artery
LMD	Local Medical Doctor
LMP	Last Menstrual Period
LN	Lymph Node
LOA	Left Occipitoanterior
LOC	Level of Consciousness
LOP	Left Occipitoposterior
LORTA	Loss of Resistance To Air
LOS	Length of Stay
Lot	Lotion
Lp	Lipoprotein
LP	Lumbar Puncture (Spinal Tap)
LPH	Left Posterior Hemiblock
LPL	Lipoprotein Lipase
LPN	Licensed Practical Nurse
LR	Lactated Ringer's Solution
LRTI	Lower Respiratory Tract Infection
LTAC	Long-term Acute Care
LSB	Left Sternal Border
LSD	Lysergic Acid Diethylamide
LUL	Left Upper Lobe-Lung
LUQ	Left Upper Quadrant
LV	Left Ventricle

	LVAD	Left Ventricular Assist Device
	LVEDP	Left Ventricular End Diastolic Pressure
	LVEF	Left Ventricular Ejection Fraction
	LVF	Left Ventricular Failure
	LVH	Left Ventricular Hypertrophy
	LVOT	Left Ventricular Outflow Track
	Ly	Lymphocytes
	lytes	Electrolytes
	L&D	Labor and Delivery (Childbirth)
	L-DOPA	Levo-Dihydroxyphenylalanine
M	M	Murmur (heart murmur)
	MAE	Moves All Extremities
	MAL	Midaxillary Line
	MAO-I	Monoamine Oxidase Inhibitor
	MAP	Mean Arterial Pressure
	MAS	Morgagni-Adams-Stokes Syndrome
	MAST	Medical Antishock Trousres
	MARSA	Methicillin and Aminoglycoside-resistant Staphylococcus aureus
	MAT	Multifocal Atrial Tachycardia
	MBT	Maternal Blood Type
	MC	Metacarpal Bone
	MCH	Mean Cell Hemoglobin
	MCH	Mean Corpuscular Hemoglobin

MCHC	Mean Cell Hemoglobin Concentration
MCP	Metacarpophalangeal Joint
MCV	Mean Cell Volume
MC&S	Microscopy, Culture and Sensitivity
MDD	Major Depressive Disorder (Clinical Depression)
MDE	Major Depressive Episode
MDI	Metered Dose Inhaler
MDS	Myelodysplastic Syndrome
MEDLINE	Medical Literature Analysis and Retrieval System Online
MEN	Multiple Endocrine Neoplasia
mEq	milliequivalent
MeSH	Medical Subject Headings
met	Metastasis
MET	Metabolic Equivalent
mg	milligram
Mg	Magnesium
MgSO4	Magnesium Sulfate
MGUS	Monoclonal Gammopathy of Undetermined Significance
MI	Myocardial Infarction (Heart Attack)
MIC	Minimum Inhibitory Concentration
MICA	Mental Illness and Chemical

	Abuse
MICU	Mobile Intensive Care Unit
MIP	Maximum Inspiratory Pressure
mL	milliliter
MLC	Mixed Lymphocyte Culture
MLE	Midline Episiotomy
MM	Myeloid Metaplasia
MMEF	Maximal Mid Expiratory Flow
mmol	millimole
MMPI	Minnesota Multiphasic Personality Inventory
MMR	Measles, Mumps, Rubella
Mo	Monocytes
mod	Moderate
mod	Modified
MODY	Maturity Onset Diabetes of the Young
MOM	Milk of Magnesia
Mono	Infectious Mononucleosis (Glandular Fever)
MOPP	Mechlorethamine, Vincristine, Procarbazine and Prednisone
MPD	Myeloproliferative Disease
MPV	Mean Platelet Volume
MR	Mitral Regurgitation
MR	Modified Release
MR	Mental Retardation

MRA	Magnetic Resonance Angiography
MRCP	Magnetic Resonance Cholangiopancreatography
MRG	Murmurs, Rubs and Gallops
MRI	Magnetic Resonance Imaging
MRSA	Methicillin-resistant Staphylococcus Aureus
MS	Multiple Sclerosis
MS	Mitral Stenosis
MS	Mental Status
MSE	Mental Status Examination
MSH	Melanocyte-Stimulating Hormone
MSM	Methylsulfonylmethane
MSSA	Methicillin-sensitive Staph aureus
MSO4	Morphine or Morphine Sulfate
MSU	Midstream Urine Sample
MSUD	Maple Syrup Urine Disease
MT	Metatarsal Bone
MTBI	Mild Traumatic Brain Injury
MTP	Metatarsalphalangeal Joint
MTX	Methotrexate
MVA	Motor Vehicle Accident
MVC	Motor Vehicle Crash
MVI	Multivitamin Injection
MVP	Mitral Valve Prolapse

	MVPS	Mitral Valve Prolapse Syndrome
	MVR	Mitral Valve Replacement
	MVV	Maximum Voluntary Ventilation
	M&M	Morbidity & Mortality
N	Na	Sodium
	NABS	Normoactive Bowel Sounds
	NAD	No Abnormality Detected
	NAD	No Apparent Distress
	NAS	No Added Salt
	NB	Newborn
	NBN	Newborn Nursery
	NC	Nasal Cannula
	NC	Nerve Action Potential
	NCC	Noncompaction Cardiomyopathy
	NCS	Nerve Conduction Study
	NCT	Nerve Conduction Test
	NCV	Nerve Conduction Velocity
	ND	Not Done
	Ne	Neutrophil Granulocytes
	NE	Norepinephrine
	NEC	Not Elsewhere Classified
	NED	No Evidence of Recurrent Disease
	Neg	Negative
	Neo	Neoplasm
	NES	Not Elsewhere Specified

NFR	Not for Resuscitation
ng	Nanogram
NG	Nasogastric
NGT	Nasogastric Tube
NGU	Non-Gonococcal Urethritis
NHL	Non-Hodgkin Lymphoma
NICU	Neonatal Intensive Care Unit
NIDDM	Non-Insulin Dependent Diabetes Mellitus (Type 2 Diabetes)
NK	Natural Killer Cells
NKA	No Known Allergies
NKDA	No Known Drug Allergies
NI	Normal
NLP	No Light Perception
NLP	Neuro-Linguistic Programming
NM	Nuclear Medicine
NMR	Nuclear Magnetic Resoance
NNH	Number Needed to Harm
NNT	Number Needed to Treat
NO	Nitric Oxide
No.	Number
NOF	Neck of Femur Fracture
Non rep.	Do not repeat
NOS	Nitric Oxide Synthase
NOS	Not Otherwise Specified
NPH	Normal Pressure Hydrocephalus
Npl	Neoplasm

NPO	Nil per os
NPTAC	No Previous Tracing Available For Comparison
NRB	Non-Rebreather Mask
NREM	Non-Rapid Eye Movement
NRM	No Regular Medications
NS	Normal Saline
NSA	No Significant Abnormality
NSAID	Non-Steroidal Anti-Inflammatory Drug
NSCC	Non-squamous-cell carcinoma
NSD	Normal Spontaneous Delivery (Natural Childbirth)
NSE	Neurospecific Enolase
NSR	Normal Sinus Rhythm
NST	Non-Stress Test
NSTEMI	Non-ST Elevation Myocardial Infarction
NSU	Non-Specific Urethritis
NT	Not Tested
NT	Nasotracheal
NTG	Nitroglycerin
NTT	Nasotracheal Tube
NVD	Normal Vaginal Delivery
NVD	Nausea, Vomiting and Diarrhea
NVDC	Nausea, Vomiting, Diarrhea and Constipation
n.s.	Not Significant

	N&V	Nausea and Vomiting
O	O2	Oxygen
	OA	Osteoarthritis
	Obl	Oblique
	OBS	Organic Brain Syndrome
	OB-GYN	Obstetrics and Gynecology
	Occ	Occasional
	OCD	Obsessive Compulsive Disorder
	OCG	Oral Cholecystogram
	OCNA	Old Chart Not Available
	OCP	Oral Contraceptive Pill
	OCPD	Obsessive Compulsive Personality Disorder
	OCT	Optical Coherence Tomography
	od	Everyday
	OD	Right Eye (Latin: Oculus Dexter)
	OD	Occupational Disease
	OD	Overdose
	OE	Otitis Externa (Ear Infection)
	OGTT	Oral Glucose Tolerance Test
	Oint	Ointment
	om	Every Morning
	OM	Otitis Media (Ear Infection)
	OME	Otitis Media with Effusion
	on	Every Night
	OOB	Out of bed

	OPD	Outpatient Department
	OPPT	Oriented to Person, Place and Time
	OPV	Outpatient Visit
	OPV	Oral Polio Vaccine
	OR	Operating Room
	ORIF	Open Reduction Internal Fixation
	ORSA	Oxacillin-resistant Staphylococcus aureus
	OS	Orthopedic Surgery
	OS	Left Eye (Ltin-Oculus Sinister)
	OSA	Obstructive Sleep Apnea
	OSH	Outside Hospital
	OSHA	Occupational Safety and Health Administration
	Osm	Osmolarity
	Osteo	Osteomyelitis
	OT	Occupational Therapy
	OTC	Over-the-counter Drug
	OTD	Out the Door
	OTPP	Oriented to Time Place and Person
	OU	Both eyes (Latin: Oculi Uterque)
	oz	Ounce
	O/E	On examination
	O&P	Ova and Parasites
P	P	Phosphorus

P	Post
P	Pulse
PA	Pulmonary Artery
PA	Posteroanterior
PA	Physician Assistant
PAC	Premature Atrial Contraction
PAC	Pulmonary Artery Catheter
PAD	Peripheral Artery Disease
PAF	Platelet Activating Factor
PAF	Paroxysmal Atrial Fibrillation
PAI-1	Plasminogen Activator Inhibitor 1
PAL	Posterior Axillary Line
PALS	Pediatric Advanced Life Support
PAN	Polyarthritis Nodosa
PAO	Peak Acid Output
PaO2	Peropheral Arterial Oxygen Content
PAO2	Alveolar Oxygen
PAOD	Peripheral Artery Occlusive Disease
Pap	Papanicolaou Test (Pap Smear)
PAP	Positive Airway Pressure
PAP	Papanicolaou Stain
PAP	Pulmonary Artery Pressure
PARA I	Indicating a woman with one child

PAT	Paroxysmal Atrial Trachycardia
PCa	Prostate Cancer
PCA	Patient Care Report
PCA	Patient-controlled Analgesia
PCD	Postconcussional Disorder
PCI	Percutaneous Coronary Intervention
PCL	Posterior Cruciate Ligament
PCN	Penicillin
PCNSL	Primary CNS Lymphoma
PCO	Polycystic Ovary
PCOS	Polycystic Ovarian Syndrome
PCP	Pneumocystis Pneumonia
PCP	Primary Care Physician
PCR	Polymerase Chain Reaction
PCS	Post-concussion Syndrome
PCV	Packed Cell Volume
PCV	Polycythemia vera
PCWP	Pulmonary Capillary Wedge Pressure
PD	Parkinson's Disease
PD	Peritoneal Disease
PDA	Patent Ductus Arteriosus
PDD	Pervasive Developmental Disorder
PDE	Phosphodiesterase
PDR	Physician's Drug Reference

PDT	Photodynamic Therapy
PE	Pre-eclampsia
PE	Pulmonary Embolism
PE	Physical Examination
PEA	Pulseless Electrical Activity
PEEP	Positive End Expiratory Pressure
PEF	Peak Expiratory Flow
PEFR	Peak Expiratory Flow Rate
PEG	Percutaneous Endoscopic Gastrostomy
pen	Penicillin
PERRL	Pupils Equal, Round, Reactive to Light
PERLA	Pupils Equal and Reactive to Light and Accomodation
Per Vag	Per Vaginam
PET	Positron-emission Tomography
PFO	Patent Foramen Ovale
PFT	Pulmonary Function Test
pg	Picogram
PGCS	Paediatric Glasgow Coma Scale
pH	Hydrogen Ion Concentration
Ph1	Philadelphia Chromosome
PH	Pulmonary Hypertension
PHx	Past History (medical)
PHTLS	Prehospital Trauma Life Support
PI	Present Illness

PI	Pulmonic Insufficiency Disease
PICC	Peripherally Inserted Central Catheter
PID	Pelvic Inflammatory Disease
PID	Prolapsed Intervertibral Disc
PIH	Pregnancy Induced Hypertension
PIP	Proximal Interphalangeal Joint
PK	Pyruvate Kinase
PKA	Protein Kinase A
PKD	Polycystic Kidney Disease
PKU	Phenylketonuria
PLAT	Tissue Plasminogen Activator
PLT	Platelets
PMB	Post-Menopausal Bleeding
PMH	Past Medical History
PMH	Perimesencephalic Subarachnoid Hemorrhage
PMI	Point of Maximal Impulse
PMN	Polymorphonuclear Leukocytes
PMS	Premenstrual Syndrome
PMR	Polymyalgia Rheumatica
PMR	Percutaneous Myocardial Revascularisation
PM&R	Physical Medicine and Rehabilitation
PND	Paroxysmal Nocturnal Dyspnea
PNM	Perinatal Mortality

POD	Postoperative Days
POEMS	Polyneuropathy, Organomegaly, Endocrinopathy, Monoclonal Protein, Skin Changes
poly	Polymorphonuclear Cells
Post	Posterior
POX	Peroxidase
PP	Post-partum
PP	Postprandial or Pulsus Paradoxus or Pulse Pressure
PPCS	Prolonged Post-Concussion Syndrome
PPD	(Cigarette) Packs Per Day
PPD	Postpartum Depression
PPD	Purified Protein Derivative or Mantoux Test
PPH	Postpartum Hemorrhage
PPH	Primary Pulmonary Hypertension
PPH	Procedure for Prolapse and Hemorrhoids
PPI	Proton Pump Inhibitor
PPROM	Preterm Premature Rupture of Membranes
Ppt	Precipitate
PPTCT	(HIV) Prevention of Parent To Child Transmission
PPTL	Post-Partum Tubal Ligation

PR	Prothrombin Ratio
PRA	Plasma Renin Activity
PRBC	Packed Red Blood Cells
Preme	Premature Baby
Prep	Preparation
PRIND	Prolonged Reversible Ischemic Neurologic Deficit
PRL	Prolactin
PRN	As Necessary
Prog	Prognosis
PROM	Premature Rupture of Membranes
PRP	PanRetinal Photocoagulation
PRV	Polycythemia rubra vera
PS	Pulmonic Stenosis
PSA	Prostate Specific Antigen
PSH	Pscychosocial History
PSP	Phenylsulphtalein
PSS	Progressive Systemic Sclerosis
PSV	Pressure Supported Ventilation
Pt	Patient
PT	Physical Therapy
PT	Prothrombin Time
PTA	Peritonsillar Abscess
PTA	Post-traumatic Amnesia
PTA	Percutaneous Transluminal Angioplasty

PTA	Prior to admission
PTB	Pulmonary Tuberculosis
PTC	Percutaneous Transhepatic Cholangiography
PTCA	Percutaneous Transluminal Coronary Angioplasty
PTD	Prior to Discharge
PTH	Parathyroid Hormone
PTHC	Percutaneous Transhepatic Cholangiography
PTSD	Post-traumatic Stress Disorder
PTSS	Posttraumatic Stress Syndrome
PTT	Partial Thromboplastin Time
PTU	Propylthiouracil
PTx	Pneumothorax
PUD	Peptic Ulcer Disease
PUO	Pyrexia of Unknown Origin
PUVA	Psoralen UV A
PVC	Premature Ventricular Contraction
PVD	Peripheral Vascular Disease
PVFS	Post-viral Fatigue Syndrome
PVR	Pulmonary Vascular Resistance
PVS	Pulmonary Valve Stenosis
PVS	Persistent Vegetative State
PWP	Pulmonary Wedge Pressure
Px	Physical Examination

	Px	Prognosis
	p.c.	After Food (Latin: Post Cibum)
	p.o.	By Mouth
	p.r.	Per rectum
	p.v.	Per Vagina
	P&A	Percussion and Auscultation
	P&PD	Percussion and Postural Drainage
	P-Y	Pack-years
Q	q	Each, every (Latin: Quaque)
	q4h, q6h	Every 4 hours, every 6 hours
	QALY	Quality-adjusted Life Years
	QNS	Quantity Not Sufficient
	QOF	Quality and Outcomes Framework
	Qs/Qt	Shunt Fraction
	qt	Quart
	Qt	Total Cardiac Output
	q.a.d.	Every Other Day (Latin: Quaque Altera Die)
	q.AM	Every morning
	q.d.	Each Day
	q.d.s.	Four Times Each Day
	q.h.	Each Hour
	q.h.s.	Every bedtime
	q.i.d.	Four Times Each Day
	q.I.	As much as you like

	q.m.t.	Every Month
	q.n.	Every Night
	q.o.d.	Every Other Day
	q.o.h.	Every other hour
	q.s.	AS much as suffices
	q.w.k.	Weekly
R	RA	Rheumatoid Arthritis
	RA	Refractory Anemia
	RA	Right Atrium
	rad	Radian
	RAD	Right Axis Deviation
	RAD	Reflex Anal Dilatation
	RAD	Reactive Attachment Disorder
	Rad hys	Radical Hysterectomy
	RAE	Right Atrial Enlargement
	RAI	Radioactive Iodine
	RAP	Right Atrial Pressure
	RAPD	Relative Afferent Pupilary Defect
	RBBB	Right Bundle Branch Block
	RBC	Red Blood Cells
	RBC	Red Blood Count
	RBP	Retino-binding Protein
	RCA	Right Coronary Artery
	RCM	Restrictive Cardiomyopathy
	RCM	Right Costal Margin
	RCT	Randomized Controlled Trial

RD	Retinal Detachment
RDA	Recommended Daily Allowance
RDS	Respiratory Distress Syndrome
RDW	Red Cell Distribution Width
RELP	Restriction Fragment Length Polymorphism
REM	Rapid Eye Movement
RES	Reticuloendothelial System
RF	Rheumatic Fever
RF	Rheumatoid Factor
RFLP	Restriction Fragment Length Polymorphism
RFT	Renal Function Test
Rh	Rhesus factor
RHD	Rheumatoid Heart Disease
RhF	Rheumatoid Factor
RIA	Radioimmunoassay
RIBA	Radioimmunoblotting Assay
RICE	Rest, Ice, Compression and Elevation
RIH	Right Inguinal Hernia
RIMA	Reversible Inhibitor of Monoamine Oxidase A
RIND	Reversible Ischemic Neurologic Deficit
RL	Ringer's Lactate
RLE	Right Lower Extremity
RLL	Right Lower Lobe-lung

RLN	Recurrent Laryngeal Nerve
RLN	Regional Lymph Node
RLQ	Right Lower Quadrant
RLS	Restless Legs Syndrome
RML	Right Middle Lobe-lung
RNA	Ribonucleioc Acid
RNV	Radionuclear Ventriculography
ROA	Right Occipital Anterior
ROM	Range of Motion
ROP	Right Occipital Posterior
ROS	Review of Systems
ROSC	Return of Spontaneous Circulation
RPG	Retrograde Pyelogram
RPR	Rapid Plasma Reagin Test
RQ	Respiratory Quotient
RR	Respiratory Rate
RRR	Regular Rate and Rhythm
RSI	Rapid Sequence Induction
RSV	Respiratory Syncytial Virus
RT	Respiratory Therapy
RTA	Renal Tubal Acidosis
RTC	Return to Clinic
RTS	Revised Trauma Source
RU	Resin Uptake
RUE	Right Upper Extremity
RUL	Right Upper Lobe - lung

	RUG	Retrograde Urethogram
	RUQ	Right Upper Quadrant
	RV	Right Ventricle
	RV	Residual Volume
	RVAD	Right Ventricular Assist Device
	RVF	Right Ventricular Failure
	RVH	Right Ventricular Hypertrophy
	RVSP	Right Ventricular Systolic Pressure
	RVT	Renal Vein Thrombosis
	Rx	Prescription Drug or medical treatment
	r/g/m	rubs/gallops/murmurs
	R/O	Rule Out
S	S	Sacrum
	S1	First Heart Sound
	S2	Second Heart Sound
	SA	Sinoatrial Node
	SAA	Syntheric Amino Acid
	SAB	Staphylococcal Bacteremia
	SAB	Spontaneous Abortion (Miscarriage)
	SAH	Subarachnoid Hemorrhage
	SAN	Sinoatrial Node
	SaO2	Oxygen Saturation of Artial Blood
	SAPS II	Simplified Acute Physiology Score

SAPS III	Simplified Acute Physiology Score
SARS	Severe Acute Respiratory Syndrome
Sat	Saturation
SB	Small Bowel
SBE	Subacute Bacterial Endocarditis
SBFT	Small Bowel Follow Through
SBO	Small Bowel Obstruction
SBP	Spontaneous Bacterial Peritonitis
SBP	Systolic Blood Pressure
SBS	Short Bowel Syndrome
SCC	Squamous Cell Carcinoma
SCID	Severe Combined Immunodeficiency
Scope	Microscope or Endoscope
SCr	Serum Creatinine
SD	Standard Deviation
SDH	Subdermal Hematoma
Sed	Sedimentation
Segs	Segmented Cells
SEM	Systolic Ejection Murmur
SFA	Serum Folic Acid
SFA	Superficial Femoral Artery
SGA	Small for Gestational Age
SGGT	Serum Gamma-Glutamyl Transpeptidase

SGOT	Serum Glutamic Oxaloacetic Transaminase
SGPT	Serum Glutamic Pyruvic Transaminase
SG cath	Swan-Ganz Catheter
SHBG	Sex Hormone-Binding Globulin
SHx	Social history
SHx	Surgical History
SI	Suicidal Ideation
SI	Seriously Ill
SI	International System of Units
SI	Sacroiliacal (SI Joint)
SIADH	Syndrome of Inappropriate Antidiuretic Hormone
SICU	Surgical Intensive Care Unit
SIDS	Sudden Infant Death Syndrome
sig	Write on label
SIMV	Synchronized Intermittent Mechanical Ventilation
SIT	Stress Inoculation Training
SK	Streptokinase
sl	Sublingual
SLE	Systemic Lupus Erythematosus
SLR	Straight Leg Raise
SM	Multiple Sclerosis
SMA	Superior Mesenteric Artery
SMA	Sequential Multiple Analysis

SMA	Spinal Muscular Atrophy
SMA-6	Six-channel Serum Multiple Analysis
SMA-7	Serum Metabolic Assay
SMO	Slips made out
SMS	Senior Medical Student
SMT	Spinal Manipulative Therapy
SMV	Superior Mesenteric Vein
SN	Student Nurse
SNB	Sentinel Node Biopsy
SNP	Sodium Nitroprusside
SNRI	Serotonin-norepinephrine Reuptake Inhibitor
SOAP	Subjective, Objective, Assessment, Plan
SOB	Shortness of Breath (Dyspnea)
SOBOE	Short of Breath On Exercise
Sol	Solution
SOL	Space Occupying Lesion
SOOB	Send Out of bed
SOS	Save Our Souls
SP	Status Post
Spec	Specimen
SPECT	Single Photon Emission Computed Tomography
SPEP	Single Protein Electrophoresis
SPET	Single Photon Emission Tomography

Sp. Fl.	Spinal Fluid
Sp. Gr.	Specific Gravity
Sq	Subcutaneous
SR	Slow Release
SROM	Spontaneous Rupture of Membranes
SS	Sickle-cell disease (anemia)
SSRI	Selective Serotonin Reuptake Inhibitor
SSS	Sick Sinus Syndrome
SSSS	Staphylococcal Sclaed Skin Syndrome
Staph	Staphylococcus
STD	Sexually Transmitted Disease
STAT	Immediately
STEMI	ST Elevation MI (Myocardial Infarction)
STH	Somatotropic Hormone
STI	Soft Tissue Injury
STI	Sexually Transmitted Infection
STNR	Symmetrical Tonic Neck Reflex
STOP	Surgical Termination of Pregnancy
Strep	Streptococcus
STS	Serological Test for Syphilis
Subq	Subcutaneous
Supp	Suppository
SV	Seminal Vesicle

	SV	Stroke Volume
	SVD	Spontaneous Vaginal Delivery
	SVI	Systemic Viral Infection
	SVN	Small Volume Nebulizer
	SVR	Systemic Vascular Resistance
	SVT	Supraventricular Tachycardia
	Sx	Symptoms
	Sx	Surgery
	SXA	Single Energy X-ray Absorptiometer
	SXR	Skull X-ray
	Sz	Seizure
	s.c.	Subcutaneous
	s.d.	Subdermal
	S&E	Sugar and Acetone
T	T	Thoracic Vertebrae
	Tab	Tablet
	TAB	Therapeutic Abortion
	TAH	Total Abdominal Hysterectomy
	TB, TBC	Tuberculosis
	TBC	Total Body Crunch
	TBG	Total Binding Globulin
	TBI	Total Body Irradiation
	TBI	Traumatic Brain Injury
	TBLC	Term Birth Living Child
	TC	Traffic Crash
	TCC	Transitional Cell Carcinoma

TCN	Tetracycline
TCT	Thrombin Clotting Time
Td	Tetanus and Diphtheria
TdP	Torsades de pointes
TEB	Thoracic Electrical Bioimpedance
TEE	Transesophageal Echocardiogram
TEM	Transmission Electron Microscopy
Temp	Temperature
TENS	Transcutaneous Electrical Nerve Stimulator
TERN	Intern
TF, T/F	Transfer
TFTs	Thyroid Function Tests
Tg	Thyroglobulin
TG	Triglycerides
TGA	Transposition of the Great Arteries
THR	Total Hip Replacement
TIA	Transient Ischemic Attack
TIBC	Total Iron Binding Capacity
Tib-Fib	Tibia and Fibula
TIG	Tetanus Immune Globulin
TIPS	Transjugular Intrahepatic Portosystemic Shunt
TKR	Total Knee Replacement

TKVO	To Keep Vein Open
TLC	Total Lung Capacity
TLC	Total Leucocyte Count
TLC	Tender Loving Care
TLR	Tonic Labyrinthine Reflex
TM	Tympanic Membrane
TM	Transcendental Meditation
TMB	Too Many Birthdays
TME	Total Mesorectal Excision
TNF	Tumor Necrosis Factors
TMJ	Temporomandibular Joint
TNG	Trinitroglycerin
TNM	Tumor-Nodes-Metastases
TNTC	Too numerous to count
TO	Telephone Order
TOA	Tuboovarian Abscess
TOD	Transoesophageal Doppler
TOE	Transoesophageal Echocardiogram
TOP	Termination Of Pregnancy (Abortion)
TOPV	Trivalent Oral Polio Vaccine
TP	Totyal Protein
TPa	Tissue Plasminogen Activator
TPN	Total Parenteral Nutrition
TPR	Temperature, Pulse, Respiration
Tr	Tincture

TR	Tricuspid Regurgitation
TRAM	Transverse Rectus Abdominis Myocutaneous Flap
TRF	Transfer
TRF'd	Transferred
TRH	Thyrotropin Releasing Hormone
TS	Tricuspid Stenosis
TSH	Thyroid Stimulating Hormone
Tsp	Teaspoon
TT	Thrombin Time
TTE	Transthoracic Echocardiogram
TTO	To Take Out
TTP	Thrombotic Thrombocytopenic Purpura
TTR	Transthyretin
TTS	Transdermal Therapeutic System
TTTS	Twin To Twin Transfusion Syndrome
Tu	Tumor
TUR	Transurethral Resection
TURBT	Transurethral Resection of Bladder Tumor
TURP	Transurethral Resection of Prostate
TV	Tridal Volume
TVH	Total Vagina Hysterectomy
tw	Twice a week
Tx	Treatment

	Tx	Transplatation (Organ Transplant)
	Tx	Traction
	t.d.s.	Three Times a day
	t.i.d.	Three times a day
	T.S.T.H.	Too sick to send home
	T&A	Tonsillectomy with Adenoidectomy
	T&C	Type and cross-match (Blood Transfusion)
	T&H	Type and Hold
U	UA	Urinalysis
	UAC	Uric Acid
	UAC	Umbilical Artery Catheter
	UAO	Upper Airway Obstruction
	UBD	Universal Blood Donor
	UBT	Urea Breath Test
	UC	Umbilical Cord
	UC	Ulcerative Colitis
	UCHD	Usual Childhood Disease
	UD	As directed
	UDS	Urine Drug Screening
	UE	Upper Extremity
	UFH	Unfractionated Heparin
	UGI	Upper Gastrointesinal
	Ung	Ointment
	Unk	Unknown

	UOP	Urinary Output
	UPJ	Ureteropelvic Junction
	URI	Upper Respiratory Infection
	URQ	Upper Respiratory Quadrant
	URTI	Upper Respiratory Tract Infection
	US	Ultrasonogram
	US	Ultrasound
	USG	Ultrasonography (Prenatal Ultrasound Imaging)
	USP	United States Pharmacopeia
	USR	Unheated Serum Reagin
	USS	Ultrasound Scan
	UTI	Urinary Tract Infection
	UUN	Urinary Urea Nitrogen
	UVAL	Ultraviolet Argon Laser
	U&E	Urea and Electrolytes
V	VA	Visual Acuity
	VAD	Ventricular Assist Device
	VAD	Venous Access Device
	VAD	Vincristine Adriblastine Dexamethasone
	Vag	Vaginal
	VAMP	Vincristine Adriblastine Methylprednisone
	VBAC	Vaginal Birth After Caesarean
	VC	Vital Capacity

vCJD	Variant Creutzfeldt-Jakob Disease
VCT	Venous Clotting Time
VCTC	Voluntary Counselling and Testing Centers
VCUG	Voiding Cysourethrogram
VD	Vaginal Delivery
VD	Volume of Distribution
VD	<u>Venereal Disease</u>
VDRF	Ventilator Dependent Respiratory Failure
VDRL	Venereal Diseases Research Laboratory
VE	Vaginal Examination
VEB	Ventricular Ectopic Beat
VF or V-fib	Ventricular Fibrillation
VIP	Vasoactive Intestinal Peptide
VLDL	Very Low Density Lipoprotein
VMA	Vanillylmandelic Acid
VMA	Violent Mechanical Asphyxia
VNPI	VanNuys Prognostic Scoring Index (Ductal Carcinoma)
VO	Verbal Order
VOD	Volume of Distribution
VPA	Valproic Acid
VPAP	Variable Positive Airway Pressure
VPB	Ventricular Premature Beats

	VPC	Ventricular Premature Contraction
	VRE	Vancomycin-Resistant Enterococcus
	VRSA	Vancomycin-resistant Staphylococcus aureus
	VS	Vital Signs
	VSD	Ventricular Septal Defect
	VSR	Ventricular Septal Rupture
	VSS	Vital Signs Stable
	VT	Ventricular tachycardia
	VTE	Venous THromboembolism
	VV	Varicose Veins
	VW	Vessel Wall
	VWD	Von Willebrand's Disease
	VZV	Varicella Zoster Virus
	V/Q	Ventilation/perfusion Scan
W	WAP	Wandering Atrial Pacemaker
	WAT	white adipose tissue
	WB	Whole Blood
	WBC	White Blood Cell, White Blood Cell Count
	WBR	whole body radiation
	WC	white cells
	WD	well developed
	WDL	within defined limits
	WDWN	well developed and well nourished

	WF	white female
	WH	Well Hydrated (no Dehydration nor Water Intoxication)
	WIA	wounded in action
	WN	well nourished
	WNL	within normal limits
	WO	written order, weeks old, wide open.
	WOP	without pain
	WPW	Wolff-Parkinson-White syndrome
	WS	Waardenburg syndrome
	WS	water-soluble
	WS	Werner syndrome
	WS	West syndrome
	WS	Wolfram syndrome
	WS	Williams Syndrome
	wt	Weight
	WWI	walking while intoxicated
	W-T-D	wet to dry
	W/	With
	w/o	without
	W/U	Workup
	W/C	Wheelchair
X	X2d	Times 2 days
	XL	Extended Release
	XL	Extra Large

	XM	Crossmatch
	XMM	Xeromammography
	XOM	Extraocular Movements
	XR	Extended Release
	XR	X-ray Radiography (Radiation Therapy)
	XRT	X-ray Threapy
	XS	Excessive
	XULN	Times Upper Limit of Normal
Y	YF	Yellow Fever
	YLC	Youngest Living Child
	YO/yo	Years Old
	YOB	Year of Birth
	ytd	Year to Date
Z	ZD	Zinc Deficiency
	ZDV	Zidovudine
	ZE	Zollinger-Ellison
	Zn	Zinc
	ZnO	Zinc Oxide
	ZIFT	Zygote Intrafallopian Transfer
	ZSB	Zero Stools Since Birth
	Z-ESR	Zeta Erythrocyte Sedimentation Rate

Common Medications

Trade Name	Generic Name	Use or Class
Dyna-Hex, Exidine-4 Scrub, BactoShield, Hibiclens Antiseptic/ Antimicrobial	Chlorhexidine Gluconate 4% in Isopropyl Alcohol 4%	Topical Antimicrobial, Topical Antiseptic
Abarelix Depot-M	Abarelix	Tx of Prostate Cancer
Abbokinase OpenCath, Abbokinase	Urokinase	Thrombolytic
Abelcet, AmBisome	Amphotericin-B Lipid Complex	Antibiotic (Polyene Antifungal)
Abilitat	Abilitat	Tx of schizophrenia
Accolate	Zafirukast	Antiasthmatic
Accupril	Quinapril HCl	Antihypertensive
Accuretic	Quinapril & Hydrochlorothiazide	Antihypertensive
AccuSite	Fluorouracil, Epinephrine & Bovine Collagen	Topical Antineoplastic
Accutane	Isotretinoin	Anti-Cystic Acne Agent
Acecol	Temocapril	Antihypertensive
Aceon	Perindopril Erbumine	Antihypertensive, ACE Inhibitor
Acidulin, Glutamic Acid HCl	Glutamic Acid HCl	Gastric Acidifier

Aciphex	Rabeprazole	Supress Gastric Acid Secretion
Aclovate	Alclometasone Dipropionate	Topical Anti-inflammatory
Acthar, ACTH	Corticotropin	Ptuitary
ActHIB, HibTITER, OmniHIB, PedvaxHIB, ProHIBit	Haemophilus B Vacciae	Vaccine
Actifed	Triprolidine& Pseudoephedrine	Antihistamine/decengestant
Actigall, URSO	Ursodiol	Urolithic
Actimmune	Interferon gamma-1b	Biologic response modifier
Actinex	Masoprocol	Tx of actinic (solar) keratoses
Actiq	Fentanyl Lozenge On A Stick	Narcotic Analgesic
Activase	Alteplase (tPA)	Thrombolytic
Activelle (Activella)	Estradiol & Norethindrone Acetate	Hormone Replacement Therapy
Actonel	Risedronate Sodium	Bone Resorption Inhibitor, Bisphosphonate
Actose	Pioglitazone HCl	Antidiabetic, (thiazolidinedione)
Acular	Ketorolac Ophthalmic	Antiinflammatory

Adagen	Pegademase Bovine	Enzyme replacement in ADA (adenosine deaminase) deficiency
Adderall	Amphetamine Aspartate/Sulfate and Dextroamphetamine Saccharate/Sulfate	CNS Stimulant
Adenocard, Adenoscan	Adenosine	Antiarrhythmic (2ml) Diagnostic Aid (30ml)
Adrenalin	Epinephrine HCl	Vasopressor, Sympathomimetic, Bronchodilator
Adrucil, 5-FU	Fluorouracil Injection	Antineoplastic
Advair Diskus	Salmeterol & Fluticasone	Antiasthmatic
Advil, Motrin, Rufen, Nuprin,Advil Chewable, Advil Migraine LiquiGel	Ibuprofen	Analgesic, Anti-inflammitory
AeroBid, Nasalide	Flunisolide	Anti-inflammitory
Aeropin	Desulfated Heparin	Tx of cystic fibrosis
Aerosporin	Polymyxin B Sulfate	Antibiotic
Afrin Tablets, Drixoral Non-Drowsy Formula	Pseudoephedrine Sulfate	Nasal Decongestant

Afrin, Allerest, Dristan Long Lasting, Genasal, Duration, Sinex Long Acting, 12 Hr Nostrilla, NTZ Long Acting Nasal, Sinarest 12-Hour, Durarist Plus	Oxymetazoline HCl Nasal	Nasal Decongestant
Aftate, Tinactin	Tolnaftate	Antifungal
Agenerase	Amprenavir	Antiviral
Aggrastat	Tirofiban	Antiplatelet
Aggrenox	Aspirin and Extended Release Dipyridamole	Antiplatelet
Aggrenox	Dipyridamole & Aspirin	Antiplatelet
Agoral Plain, Kondremul	Mineral Oil Emulsion	Laxative
Agrylin	Anagrelide HCl	Platelet Reducing Agent
AK Tracin	Bacitracin Ophth. Oint.	Ophth. Antibacterial
AK-Cide, Metimyd, Ocu-Lone,	Sulfacetamide & Prednisolone	Ophth. Antibacterial, Antiinflammatory
Akineton	Biperiden	Anticholinergic, Antiparkinson

Akne-Mycin, A/T/S Gel, A/T/S Sol, Emgel, Erycette, EryDerm, Erythra Derm Sol, Erythrostatin Sol, Staticin Sol, T-Stat Pads, Theramycin Z Sol, T-Stat Sol, Erygel	Erythromycin Topical	Topical antibiotic
Alagesic, Americet, Anolor 300, Arcet, Esgic, Esgic Plus, Endelor,Ezol, Fioricet, Fiorpap, Geone, Margesic, Medigesic, Minetal, Nonbac, Pacaps, Pharmagesic, Repan, Tenake, Tencet, Triad, Zebutal	Acetaminophen, Butalbital & Caffine	Analgesic/Antipyretic
Alamast	Pemirolast	Tx of allergic conjunctivitis
Ala-Quin, Corque, Dek-Quin, Steroform	Clioquinol and Hydrocortisone	Antiinflammatory and Antifungal
Albamycin	Novobiocin	Antibiotic
Albenza, Zentel, Valbazen,	Albendazole	Anthelminic, Hydatid Disease

Eskazole		
Albuminar, Buminate, Albumarc	Albumin	Plasma Volume Expander
Alcar, Acetyl Levocarnitine	Acetylcarnitine	Adjunct in the Tx of Alzheimer's
Aldactazide	Hydrochlorothiazide and Spironolactone	Diuretic
Aldactazide	Spironolactone and Hydrochlorothiazide	Combination Diuretic
Aldactone	Spironolactone	Diuretic
Aldara	Imiquimod	Immune response modifier
Aldochlor-250	Methyldopa and Chlorothiazide	Antihypertensive
Aldomet	Methyldopa	Antihypertensive
Aldomet	Methyldopate HCl	Antihypertensive
Aldoril-D50, Aldoril-15, Aldoril-D30, Aldoril-25	Methyldopa and Hydrochlorothiazide	Antihypertensive
Aldurazyme	Recombinant a-L-Iduronidase	Tx of musopolysacchridosis-I
Aleve Cold & Sinus	Naproxen Sodium & Pseudoephedrine	Analgesic and decongestant
Aleve, Anaprox	Naproxen, Sodium	Analgesic, Antiinflammatory

Alfenta	Alfentanil HCl	Analgesic, Anesthetic-narcotic
Alferon-N	Interferon Alfa-n3	Tx of genital or venereal warts
Alibra	Alprostadil & Prazosin	Tx of Erectile Dysfunction
Aliminase	Acetylated Carbohydrate	Tx of ulcerative colitis
Alimta	Pemetrexed Disodium	Tx of advanced cancers
Alkeran	Melphalan	Antineoplastic
Allegra	Fexofenadine HCl	Non-Sedating Antihistamine
Allegra-D	Fexofenadine HCl and Pseudoephedrine	Non-Sedating Antihistamine and Decongestant Combo.
Allervax Cat	Antihypertensive Cat Allergen	Tx of atopic individuals allergic to cat dander
Allovectin-7	DNA-lipid complex encoding HLA-B7 antigen	Tx of metastatic melanoma, head and neck squamous cell carcinoma
Alocril	Nedocromil Sodium Ophthalmic Solution	Ophth. Antiinflammatory
Alomide	Lodoxamide Tromethamine Ophth	Antiallergic
Alpha Tocopherol	Vitamin E	Vitamin
Alphagan	Brimonidine	Antiglaucoma
Alredase	Tolrestat	Aldose reductase

		inhibitor
Altace	Ramipril	Antihypertensive
Altropane	I-123 Imaging Agent	Dx of Parkinson's Disease
Aluminum Paste	Aluminum Ointment	Occlusive Skin Protectany
Alupent, Metaprel	Metaproterenol Sulfate	Bronchodilator
Amaryl	Glimepiride	Antidiabetic
Ambien	Zolpidem	Hypnotic, sedative
Amdray	Valspodar	Antineoplastic
Amerge	Naratriptan	Antimigraine
Americaine, Hurricaine, Dermoplast	Benzocaine	Topical Anesthetic
Amevive	Alefacept	Tx of psoriasis
Amicar	Aminocaproic Acid	Systemic Hemostatic
Amidate	Etomidate	General Anesthetic
Amikin	Amikacin Sulfate	Antibiotic
Amipaque	Metrizamide	Diagnostic Aid
Amisdyl	Amsacrine	Tx of Acute Leukemia and Lymphoma
Amlactin	Lactic Acid Cream	Moisturizing Cream
Ammonium Chloride	Ammonium Chloride	Urinary Acidifier
Amoxil, Polymox, Biomox, Wymox, Alphamox, Cilamox, Moxacin, Novamoxin	Amoxicillin Trihydrate	Antibiotic

Amphojel	Aluminum Hydroxide Gel	Antacid
Amphotec	Amphotericin B Cholesteryl Sulfate Complex	Antibiotic (Polyene Antifungal)
Ampligen	Atvogen	'Interferon Inducer'
Amsacrine	Acridinyl Anisidide	Antineoplastic
Amytal	Amobarbital Sodium	Hypnotic, Sedative
Anadrol-50	Oxymetholone	Anabolic Steroid
Anafranil	Clomipramine	Antidepressant
Anatrast	Barium Sulfate Paste	Diagnostic Aid
Ancef, Kefzol, Zolicef	Cefazolin	Antibiotic
Ancobon, Ancotil	Flucytosine	Antifungal
Andractim, DHT	Dihydrotestosterone	Tx of AIDS related wasting syndrome
Androderm, Testoderm TTS, Testoderm	Testosterone Transdermal	Tx of hypogonadism in men
AndroGel	Testosterone Gel	Tx of hypogonadism in men
Androlone-D, Deca-Durabolin, Neo-Durabolic, Hybolin Decanoate, Neo-Durabolic	Nandrolone Decanoate	Anabolic Steroid
Angio Conray	Iothalamate Sodium 80%	Diagnostic Aid

Angiomax, Hirulog	Bivalirudin	Hirudin, Thrombin Inhibitor-Anticoagulant
Angiovist 282, Mypaque Meglumine 60%, Reno-M-60	Diatrizoate Meglumine 60%	Diagnostic Aid
Angiovist 292, MD-60, Renografin-60	Diatrizoate Meglumine 55% and Diatrizoate Sodium 8%	Diagnostic Aid
Angiovist 370, Hypaque-76, MD-76, Renografin-76	Diatrizoate Meglumine 66% and Diatrizoate Sodium 10%	Diagnostic Aid
Ansaid, Froben	Flurbiprofen	Analgesic, Antiinflammitory
Antabuse	Disulfiram	Alcohol Abuse Deterrent
Antagon	Ganirelix	Hormone supression. Gonadotropin releasing hormone antagonist.
Antegren	Natalizumab	Tx of Multiple Sclerosis, Tx of Crohn's Disease
Anthra-Derm, Dritrocream, Anthrascalp	Anthralin	Antipsoriatic
Anti-IgE, rhuMAb-E25	Olizumab	Monoclonal antibody
Antilirium	Physostigmine Salicylate	Antidote, Cholinesterase

		Inhibitor
Antivenin (crotalidae) Polyvalent, CroTAB	Rattlesnake Antivenin	Antivenin
Antivert, Bonine, Medivert, Meni-D, Bonamine	Meclizine	Antiemetic,Antivertigo
Antizol	Femepizole (4-Methylpyrazole, 4-MP)	Antidote
Antocin	Atosiban	Antagonist at oxytocin receptors
Antrocol Elixir	Atropine & Phenobarbital Liguid	GI-Antichohinergic, Antispasmotic
Anturane	Sulfinpyrazone	Uricosuric
Anusol, Fleet Pain Relief, ProctoFoam NS	Pramoxine, Zinc Oxide, Mineral Oil	Tx of hemorroids
Anusol-HC, Corticaine, Cortifoam, Cortaid, Orabase-HCA	Hydrocortisone Acetate Topical	Topical Antiinflammatory
Anusol-HC,Cort-Dome, Proctocream-HC, Hytone, Cortizone, Hycort, Tegrin HC, Dermolate,	Hydrocortisone Topical	Topical Antiinflammatory

Synacort, Cortoderm		
Anzemet	Dolasetron Mesylate	Antiemetic
Aphrodyne, Yohimex, Dayto Himbin, Yocon, Actibine	Yohimbine HCl	Tx of erectile dysfunction
Aphthasol Oral Paste	Amlexanox	Antiinflammatory
APL, Pregnyl, Chorex, Profasi, HCG Injection, Novarel, Choron, Gonic	Chorionic Gonadotropin	Ovulation Induction
Apligraf	Graftskin	Tx of diabetic foot ulcers
Apresazide	Hydralazine and Hydrochlorothiazide	Ahtihypertensive
Apresoline	Hydralazine HCl	Peripheral Vasodialator
Aptosyn	Exisulind	Antineoplastic
Aqua-Ban	Ammonium Chloride & Caffeine	Diuretic
Aqua-Ban Plus	Ammonium Chloride, Caffeine & Ferrous Sulfate	Diuretic

Aquacare, Nutraplus, Carmol 20, Gormel Cream, Lanaphillic, Ureacin-20, Gordon's Urea 40%	Urea (Carbamide) Cream	Promote hydration, keratolytic
Aquatensen, Enduron	Methyclothiazide	Thiazide Diuretic
Aralen Phosphate with Primaquine Phosphate	Chloroquine with Primaquine	Antimalarial
Aralen, Chlorquin, Avlocor	Chloroquine Phosphate	Antimalarial
Aramine	Metaraminol Bitartrate	Vasopressor, Symphathomimetic
ARANESP	Darbepoetin Alfa (NESP, Novel Erythropoiesis Stimulating Protein)	Stimuate red blood cell production
Arava	Leflunomide	Rheumatoid Arthritis
Arduan	Pipecuronium Bromide	Muscle Relaxant
Aredia	Pamidronate Disodium	Bisphosphonate
Arestin	Minocycline Microsphere injection	Antibiotic
Arfonad	Trimethaphan Camsylate	Antihypertensive

Aricept	Donepezil	Treatment of Alzheimer's Disease
Arimidex	Anastrozole	Aromatase Inhibitor
Aristocort Intralesional, Trilone, Amcort, Aristocort Forte, Tristoject, Clinacort	Triamcinolone Diacetate	Anti-inflammatory
Aristospan Intralesional, Aristospan Intra-Articular	Triamcinolone Hexacetonide	Anti-inflammatory
Arixtra	Fondaparinux (SR90107) (Pentasaccharide)	Antithrombotic.
Arkin-Z	Vesnarinone	Tx of CHF
Arlidin	Nylidrin	Peripheral Vasodilator
Aromasin	Exemestane	Antineoplastic
Arsobal	Melarsoprol (Mel B)	Anttinfective
Artane, Aparkane	Trihexyphenidyl	Antiparkinson, Anticholinergic
Arthropan	Choline Salicylate	Anti-inflammatory, Analgesic
Arthrotec	Diclofenac Sodium & Misoprostol	Antiinflammatory, Analgesic
Ascorbic Acid	Vitamin C	Vitamin
Ascriptin, Bufferin	Aspirin, Buffered	Analgesic, Antipyretic
Asendin	Amoxapine	Antidepressant

Aslera, GL701	Prasterone (Dehydroepiandrost erone)	Tx of systemic lupus
Aslera, GL701, DHEA	Dehydroepiandrost erone (Prasterone)	Tx of systemic lupus
Astelin	Azelastine Nasal	Antihistamine
AsthmaNefrin, S-2, MicroNefrin, Nephron	Epinephrine Racemic Mixture (Racepinephrioe)	Tx of severe croup
Astramorph-PF, Duramorph, Statex, MS-Contin, Roxanol, Oramorph-SR, Kadian, MS-Contin, MSIR, MS/L	Morphine Sulfate	Narcotic analgesic
Atabrine HCl	Quinacrine HCl	Anthelminic, Antimalarial
Atacand	Candesartan	Antihypertensive
Atacand-HCT	Candesartan and Hydrochlorothiazid e	Antihypertensive
Atarax, Vistaril Inj.	Hydroxyzine HCl	Sedative, Antipruitic, Antianxiety, Antiemetic
Ativan	Lorazepam	Anxiolytic, Antiseizure
Atragen	Tretinoin, Liposomal	Antineoplastic
Atridox	Doxycycline 10%	Tx of chronic adult periodontitis

Atromid-S	Clofibrate	Antilipemic
Atropine	Atropine	Tx of bradyarrhythmia/CPR
Atrovent	Ipratropium Bromide	Bronchodilator
Augmentin, Clavulin	Amoxicillin & Potassium Clavulanate	Antibiotic
Auralgan	Antipyrine & Benzocaine	Otic Analgesic, Cerumenolytic,
Aureomycin	Chlortetracycline	Antibiotic
Aurorix	Aurorix	Tx of social anxiety disorder
Avalide	Irbesartan and Hydrochlorothiazide	Antihypertensive
Avandia	Rosiglitazone	Antidiabetic, (thiazolidinedione)
Avapro	Irbesartan	Antihypertensive
AVC, Vagitrol	Sulfanilamide	Antibacterial
Aveeno	Oatmeal	Tx of pruritus from poison oak/ivy
Avelox	Moxifloxacin	3rd Gen Quinolone Antibiotic
Aventyl, Pamelor	Nortriptyline HCl	Antidepressant
Avitene	Collagen Microfibrilar Hemostat	Hemostatic
Avonex	Interferon Beta-1a	For Multiple Sclerosis
Avosulfon,	Dapsone	Leprostatic,

Dapsone		Antiprotazoan
Axert	Almotriptan Maleate	Tx of migraine
Axid	Nizatidine	H2 Antagonist
Aygestin, Norlutate	Norethindrone Acetate	Progestin
Azacitidine	Ladakamycin, 5-AZC, AZA-CR, 5-Azacytidine	Antineoplastic
Azactam	Aztreonam	Antibiotic
Azelex, Finevin	Azelaic Acid	Tx of acne
Azlin	Azlocillin	Antibiotic
Azo-Gantrisin, Azo-Sulfisoxazole	Sulfisoxazole and Phenazopyridine HCl	Antibiotic, urinary analgesic combination
Azopt	Brinzolamide Ophth. Susp.	Antiglaucoma
Azo-Sulfisoxazole, Azo-Gantrisin	Phenazopyridine and Sulfisoxazole	Urinary antibiotic and Urinary Analgesic
Aztec, AZT	Zidovudine extended release	Antiviral
Azulfidine, S.A.S., Azulfidine EN-tabs, Salazopyrin EN-tabs	Sulfasalazine	Antiinflammatory
B&O Suppositories	Belladonna & Opium Suppositories	Opiate Agonist
B.S.S.	Balanced Salt Ophthalmic Solution	EENT Miscellaneous

Bacid, Lactinex, Intestinex, Probiotica	Lactobacillus	Antidiarrheal
Baciguent, Bacitracin Ointment	Bacitracin Topical	Topical antiinfective
Bactoshield	Chlorhexidine Gluconate 4% and Isopropyl Alcohol 4% Foam	Topical Antimicrobial, Topical Antiseptic
BactoShield, Exidine-2 Scrub, Dyna-Hex-2, Bactoshield	Chlorhexidine Gluconate 2% in Isopropyl Alcohol 4%	Topical Antimicrobial, Topical Antiseptic
Bactrim, Septra	Cotrimoxazole Injection	Antibiotic
Bactrim, Septra (Cotrimoxizole)	Trimethoprim & Sulfamethoxazole	Antibiotic (Sulfa)
Bactrim, Septra, Sulfatrim, Cotrim, TMP/SMX	Cotrimoxazole Oral	Antibiotic
Bactrim, Septra, Sulfatrim, Cotrim, TMP/SMX	Sulfamethoxazole & Trimethoprim	Antibiotic
Bactroban	Mupirocin (Pseudomonic Acid A)	Topical Antibiotic
BAL in Oil	Dimercaprol	Antidote
Banana Bag, Rally Pack	Thiamine, MgSO4, and Multivitamins I.V.	Dietary supplement in alcoholic malnutrition.

Barium Sulfate USP, Baroflave	Barium Sulfate Powder	Diagnostic Aid
Baro-Cat, Prepac, Enecat, Tomocat, Emtrobar, Liquid Barosperse, HD 85, Barobag, Lipipake, Flo-Coat, Epi-C	Barium Sulfate Suspension	Diagnostic Aid
Baycol	Cerivastatin	Antihyperlipidemic
Baypress	Nitrendipine	Type II calcium channel blocker
BCI Immune Activator	Keyhole Limpet Hemocyanin, Modified	N/A
Beclovent, Vanceril, Vanceril-DS, QVAR	Beclomethasone Dipropionate MDI	Anti-inflammatory
Beconase, Vancenase	Beclomethasone Dipropionate Nasal	Anti-inflammatory
Beconase-AQ	Beclomethasone Dipropionate, Monohydrate	Anti-Inflammatory
Beesix, Nestrex, Vitamin B6	Pyridoxine HCl (Vitamin B-6)	Vitamin
Bel-Phen-Ergot SR, Bellacane SR	L-Alkaloids of Belladonna, Phenobarbital and Ergotamine Tartrate Sustained Release	GI-Antichohinergic, Antispasmotic
Benadryl Cream	Diphenhydramine Topical	Antipruritic, Topical Anesthetic

Benadryl, Banophen, Diphenhist, AllerMax, Nighttime Sleep Aid, Diphen AF, Genahist, Scot-Tussin Allergy DM, Siladryl, Tusstat, Hyrexin-50, Allerdryl, Aleernix, Nytol, Midol PM, Snooze Fast, 40 Winks, Dormin, Miles Nervine, Sominex, Sleepwell 2-night, Dtuss, Excedrine PM, Truxadryl, Bantril, Benoject-10, Wehdryl-50	Diphenhydramine HCl	Antihistamine, Antiemetic, Antiparkinson Agent
Benemid, Benuryl	Probenecid	Uricosuric
Benilas	Oxaprozin Potassium	Fast acting NSAID, Analgesic
Benoquin	Monobenzone	Skin Bleach
Bentyl, Antispas, Bentylol	Dicyclomine HCl	Anticholinergic
BenzaClin Topical Gel	Clindamycin and Benzoyl Peroxide	Tx of acne
Benzedrex	Propylhexedrine	Decongestant
Beriplast HS, Beriplast-S	Fibrin Sealant	Hemostatic

Berotec	Fenoterol HBr	Bronchodilator
Beta LT, Betathine	Beta Alethine	Immune system stimulant
Betadine	Povidone-Iodide Shampoo	Antiseborrheic
Betadine Ophth.	Povidone Iodine Ophth.	Antiseptic Preparation
Betadine, Betagen, Etodine, Iodex, Mallisol, Minidyne, Operand, Povidine, Polydine	Povidone Iodine	Antiseptic Preparation
Betafectin	Beta-Glucan, Recombinant	Glucose Polymer
Betagan Liquifilm	Levobunolol	Antiglaucoma
Betalin-S	Thiamine (Vit.B-1)	Vitamin
Betapace, Rylosol, Betapace AF, Sotacar, Sorine	Sotalol HCl	Group III Antiarrhythmic, ß-Adrenergic Blocker
Betapen-VK, Beepen-VK, Pen-V, Ledercillin-VK, Pen-Vee K, V-Cillin-K, Veetids	Penicillin-V Potassium (Phenoxymethyl Penicillin)	Antibiotic
Betaseron	Interferon Beta-1b	For Multiple Sclerosis
Betaxon	Levobetaxolol HCl	Antiglaucoma Agent
Betoptic, Betoptic-S	Betaxolol Ophth. Sol.	Antiglaucoma agent
Bextra	Bucindolol	Beta Blocker

Bexxar	Tositumemab/Iodine I-131 Tositumomab	Antineoplastic
Biaxin, Biaxin XL	Clarithromycin	Antibiotic
Bicillin-CR	Penicillin-G Benzathine and Penicillin-G Procaine	Antibiotic
Bicillin-LA, Permapen	Penicillin-G Benzathine	Antibiotic
Bicitra, Oracit	Sodium Citrate & Citric Acid	Alkalinizing Agent
BiCNU, BCNU, Gliadel Wafer	Carmustine	Antineoplastic
Bilivist, Oragrafin Sodium	Ipodate Sodium	Diagnostic Aid
Bilopaque	Tyropanoate Sodium	Diagnostic Aid
Biltricide	Praziquantel	Anthelmintic
Bisolvon	Bromhexine	Tx of mild/moderate kertoconjunctivitis sicca in Sjögren's Syndrome
Blenoxane	Bleomycin Sulfate	Antineoplastic
Bleph-10, Sodium Sulamyd, Klaron, Isopto Cetamide, Sulfair, Sebizon	Sulfacetamide Sodium	Antiinfective

Blocadren	Timolol Tablets	Beta Blocker, Antiarrhythmic, Antihypertensive, Antimigraine
BNP	Brain-Type Natriuretic Peptide	Tx of acutely decompensated CHF
Bonefos	Clodronate Tetrahydrate	Bisphosphonate
Bonviva (IV & oral), Bondronat (IV), Bondronate	Ibandronate	Bone Resorption Inhibitor, Bisphosphonate
Botox	Botulinum Toxin, Type A	Tx of strabismus, blepharospasm, cervical dystonia
Bradycor	Deltibant	Tx of severe systemic inflammatory response in pts with sepsis
Brethine, Bricanyl	Terbutaline Sulfate	Bronchodilator also to delay premature lagor
Bretylol, Bretylate	Bretylium Tosylate	Antiarrhythmic
Brevibloc	Esmolol HCl	ß-Blocker, Group II Antiarrhythmic
Brevital Sodium	Methohexital Sodium	Barbiturate Anesthetic
Brolene	Propamidine isothionate ophthalmic	Acanthamoeba keratitis
Brondelate Elixir	Oxtriphylline and Guaifenesin Elixer	Bronchodialator, Expectorant

Bronkaid Mist Susp., Primatine Mist Susp.	Epinephrine Bitartrate	Bronchodilator
Bronkometer, Bronkosol	Isoetharine HCl	Bronchodilator
Broxine, BUdR	Broxuridine	Radiation sensitizer in the Tx of primary brain tumor
Bucladin-S	Buclizine HCl	Antiemetic, Antivertigo
Buffets II Tablets	APAP, Aspirin, Caffeine and Aluminum Hydroxide	Analgesic
Bumex	Bumetanide	Diuretic
Buphenyl	Sodium Phenylbutyrate	Prodrug used to treat urea cycle disorders
Buprenex, Subutex	Buprenorphine	Analgesic, Opiate partial agonist
Buspar	Buspirone	Anxiolytic
BuSpar Patch	Buspirone HCl Topical	Anxiolytic
Busulfex, Spartaject	Busulfan Injection	Antineoplastic
Butibel, Butibel Elixir	Belladonna Alkaloids & Butibarbital	GI-Antichohinergic, Antispasmotic
Butisol	Butabarbital	Hypnotic, sedative
Cachexon	Reduced L-glutathione	AIDS-associated cachexia
Cafcit	Caffeine Citrate	CNS Stimulant

Cafergot, Cafatine, Catetrate, Wigraine	Ergotamine Tartrate and Caffeine Supp.	Antimigraine
Caladryl Lotion	Calamine, Diphenhydramine Lotion	Topcal Emollient, Protectant
Calamine Lotion	Calamine	Topcal Emollient, Protectant
Calan, Isoptin, Verelan, Covera-HS	Verapamil	Group IV Antiarrhythmic, Calcium Channel Blocker, Antianginal, Antihypertensive
Calciferol	Vitamin D	Vitamin
Calciferol, Deltalin, Drisdol, Vitamin-D	Ergocalciferol	Vitamin
Calcijex, Rocaltrol, Vitamin D	Calcitriol	Hypocalcemia, hypoparathyroidism, Hypophosphatemia
Calcimar	Calcitonin-Salmon Injection	Parathyroid, Treatment of Paget's Disease, Hypercalcemia, Osteoporosis
Calcium Chloride Injection	Calcium Chloride	Calcium
Calcium Disodium Versenate	Edetate Calcium Disodium (Calcium EDTA)	Antidote
Calcium Gluconate Injection	Calcium Gluconate	Calcium

Calcium Gluconate Tablets	Calcium Gluconate	Calcium Suppliment
Calcium Lactate	Calcium Lactate	Calcium Suppliment
Campath	Alemtuzumab	Tx of B-cell refractory lymphocytic leukemia
Campral	Acamprosate (Calcium Acetylhomotaurinate)	Tx of alcoholsim
Camptogen, 9-nitro-camptothecin	Rubitecan	Antineoplastic
Camptosar, CPT-11	Irinotecan	Antineoplasic
Campyvax	Campylobacter Vaccine	Vaccine
Canasa, Fivasa	Mesalamine Supp.	Tx of active ulcerative proctitis
Cancidas	Caspofungin Acetate	Antifungal
Cantil	Mepenzolate Bromide	GI Anticholinergic, Antispasmotic
Capastat	Capreomycin	Antibiotic, Antituberculosis agent
Capitrol	Chloroxine	Antibacterial
Capoten	Capopril	Antihypertensive
Capozide	Captopril, Hydrochlorothiazide	Antihypertensive
Caprogel	Aminocaproic Acid Topical	Topical Tx of traumatic hyphema of the eye

Carafate	Sucralfate	Gastric Protectant
Carbinoxamine Compound Drops	Carbinoxamine, Pseudoephedrine & Dextromethorphan Drops	Antihistamine, Decongestant & Antitussive
Carbinoxamine Compound Syrup, Cardec-DM Syrup, Rondec-DM Syrup, Tussafed Syrup, Pseudo-Car DM Syrup	Carbinoxamine, Pseudoephedrine & Dextromethorphan	Antihistamine, Decongestant & Antitussive
Carbinoxamine Syrup, Rondec Syrup, Cardec Syrup	Carbinoxamine & Pseudoephedrine	Antihistamine & Decongestant
Carbiset, Carbodec, Rondec	Carbinoxamine & Pseudoephedrine	Antihistamine & Decongestant
Carbocaine, Polocaine	Mepivacaine HCl	Local Anesthetic
Cardene	Nicardipine HCl	Calcium Channel Blocker, Antianginal, Antihypertensive
Cardioquin	Quinidine Polygalacturonate	Group I-A Antiarrhythmic
Cardizem, Tiazac, Dilacor-XR, Cartia-XT, Cardizem-CD, Taztia XT, Cardizem-SR, Diltia XT, Tiamate	Diltiazem HCl	Calcium Channel Blocker, Antianginal, Antihypertensive

Cardura	Doxazosin Mesylate	Antihypertensive, Benign Prostatic Hyperplasia (BPH)
Carmol 10, Aquacare, Nutraplus, Ureacin-10, Ultra Mide 25	Urea (Carbamide) Lotion	Promote hydration, keratolytic
Carnitor	Levocarnitine	Vitamin Suppliment
Cartrol	Carteolol HCl	ß-Adrenergic Blocker, Antihypertensive
Casodex	Bicalutamide	Non-steroidal Antiandrogen
Cataflam	Diclofenac Potassium	Analgesic, Antiinflammatory
Catapres, Dixaril	Clonidine	Antihypertensive
Catapress-TTS	Clonidine Patches	Antihypertensive
Catatrol	Viloxazine	Antidepressant
Caverject, Edex, Muse	Alprostadil (PGE1 Prostaglandin E1)	Tx of erectile dysfunction
Ceclor	Cefaclor	Antibiotic
Cedax	Ceftibuten	Antibiotic
CeeNu, CCNU	Lomustime	Antineoplastic
Cefadyl	Cephapirin	Antibiotic
Cefizox	Ceftizoxime	Antibiotic
Cefmax	Cefmenoxime	Antibiotic, Cephalosporin III
Cefobid	Cefoperazone	Antibiotic
Cefotan	Cefotetan	Antibiotic
Ceftin	Cefuroxime Axetil	Antibiotic

Cefzil	Cefprozil	Antibiotic
Celebrex	Celecoxib	Anti-inflammatory, analgesic, NSAID (COX-2 Inhibitor)
Celestone Phosphate, Cel-U-Jec	Betamethasone Sodium Phosphate	Adrenal Steroid, Glucocorticoid
Celestone Soluspan	Betamethasone Sodium Phosphate and Betamethasone Acetate	Adrenal Steroid, Glucocorticoid
Celestone, Beben	Betamethasone	Adrenal Steroid, Glucocorticoid
Celexa	Citalopram	Antidepressant
CellCept	Mycophenolate Mofetil	Immunosupressant
Celontin Kapseals	Methsuximide	Anticonvulsant
Cenestin	Synthetic Conjugated Estrogen A	Estrogen
Centoxin	Nebacumab	G- endotoxic shock
Centrax	Prazepam	Sedative
CerAxon	Citicoline	Oral agent for management of ischemic stroke
Cerebrolysin	Cerebrolysin	Neuroprotective agent for Tx of Alzheimer's
Cerebyx	Fosphenytoin	Anticonvulsant
Ceredase	Algluccrase	Replacement therapy in Gaucher's Disease

Ceresine, CPC-211	Sodium Dichloroacetate	Tx of lactic acidosis
Cerestat	Aptiganel	Ion-channel blocking agent
Cerezyme	Imiglucerase	Treatment of Gaucher's Disease
Cerumenex	Triethanolamine Otic	Otic
Cetrotide	Cetrorelix Acetate	Hormone supression. Gonadotropin releasing hormone antagonist
CharcoCaps, Charcoal, Charcoal Plus, Actidose Actichar, CharcoAid, Charcodate, acitvated charcoal	Charcoal	Detoxicant, Gastric adsorbent
Chelated Magnesium	Magnesium Amino Acids Chelate	Replacement Preparation
Chemet	Succimer	Tx of lead poisoning
Chenenodeoxycholic acid, Chenix	Chenodiol	Gallstones
Chibroxin	Norfloxacin Ophth.	Antibiotic
Chirocaine	Levobupivacaine	Local Anesthetic
ChloraPrep, Hibiclens, Dyna-Hex, Exidine, Hibiscrub, Hibistat	Chlorhexidine Gluconate Topical	Topical Antiinfective
Chloromycetin	Chloramphenicol	Antibiotic

Chloromycetin Cream	Chloramphenicol Topical	Topical Antibiotic
Chloromycetin Otic	Chloramphenicol. Otic Solution	Otic Anti-infective
Chloroptic	Chloramphenicol Ophthalmic	Ophth. Antibiotic
Chlor-Trimeton, Teldrin, Aller-Chlor, Chlo-Amine, Allergy	Chlorpheniramine	Antihistamine
Cholebrine	Iocetamic Acid	Diagnostic Aid
Cholecalciferol	Vitamin D3	Vitamin
Choledyl	Oxtriphylline	Bronchodialator
Cholera Vaccine	Cholera Vaccine	Vaccine
Cholografin Meglumine	Iodipamide Meglumine 10.3%	Diagnostic Aid
Cholografin Meglumine	Iodipamide Meglumine 52%	Diagnostic Aid
Choloxin	Dcxtrothyroxinc Sodium	Antihyperlipidemic
Chromelin Complexion Blender	Dihydroxyacetone	Skin Bleach
Chronulac, Cephulac, Duphalac, Enulose, Acilac	Lactulose Syrup	Ammonia Detoxicant, Laxative
Chymodiactin	Chymopapain	Pryteolytic Enzyme
Cialis	IC351	For Diabetic Related Erectile Dysfunction

Cibacalcin	Calcitonin-Human	Paget's disease (Orphan Drug)
Cidecin IV	Daptomycin	Antibacterial
Ciloxan	Ciprofloxacin Ophthalmic	Ophthalmic Antibiotic
Cinobac	Cinoxacin	Urinary Antiinfective
Cipralan, Cibenzoline	Cifenline Succinate (formerly Cibenzoline)	Antiarrhythmic
Cipro	Ciprofloxacin	Quinolone Antibiotic
Cipro-HC Otic	Ciprofloxacin and Hydrocortisone Otic Suspension	Otic Preparation
Cisto-Conray II (not intended for intravascular admin)	Iothalamate Meglumine 17,2%	Diagnostic Aid
Citanest	Prilocaine	Local Anesthetic
Citracal	Calcium Citrate	Calcium Suppliment
Citrolith	Potassium Citrate & Sodium Citrate	Urinary Alkalinizer
Citroma	Magnesium Citrate Solution	Saline Laxative
Claforan	Cefotaxime	Antibiotic
Clarinex	Desloratadine	Non-Sedating Antihistamine
Claritin	Loratadine	Non-Sedating Antihistamine
Claritin D	Loratadine and Pseudoephedrine	Non-Sedating Antihistamine and Decongestant combo.

Cleocin Vaginal, Dalacin	Clindamycin Vaginal	Antibacterial
Cleocin, Dalacin C	Clindamycin	Antibiotic
Cleocin-T, Clindets 1% Dalactin-T	Clindamycin Topical	Anti-Acne Agent, Topical Antibiotic
Clinoquinol, Vioform	Iodochlorhydroxyquin	Topical Antifungal
Clinoril	Sulindac	Antiinflammatory, Analgesic
Cloderm	Clocortolone Pivalate	Corticosteroid, Anti-Inflammatory
Clomid, Serophene, Milophene	Clomiphene Citrate	Fertility Agent
Cloxapen, Tegopen, Orbenin, Orbenin	Cloxacillin	Antibiotic
Clozaril	Clozapine	Antipsychotic
Coactinon, MKC-442	Emivirine	Antiretroviral
Codeine	Codeine	Opioid analeesic
Cogentin, Bensylate	Benztropine Mesylate	Antiparkinson, Anticholinergic
Cognex	Tacrine HCl	Treatment of Alzheimer's Disease
Colace, Diocto, DSS, Dialose	Docusate Sodium	Stool Softener
Colazal, Balasa, Colazide	Balsalazide Disodium	Tx of ulcerative colitis
ColBenemid	Colchicine &	Uricosuric Agent

	Probenecid	
Colchicine	Colchicine	Tx of acute gouty arthritis
Colestid	Colestipol	Antilipemic Agent
Colymycin-M	Colistimethate Sodium (Colistin, Polymyxin-E)	Antibiotic
Colymycin-S	Colistin, Hydrocortisone, Neomycin and Thonzonium	Otic Antibiotic, Antiinflammatory
Combidex	Ferumoxtran-10	MRI Contrast Media
CombiPatch	Estradiol & Norethindrone Acetate Transdermal	Hormone Replacement Therapy
Combipres, Clorpres	Clonidine and Chlorthalidone	Antihypertensive
Combisor	Mometasone Furoate and Salicylic Acid	Tx of psoriasis
Combivent, Duovent	Ipratropium and Albuterol Inhaler	Bronchodilator Anticholinergic combination
Combivir	Zidovudine & Limivudine	Antiviral
Compazine, Stemetil, Compro	Prochlorperazine	Antiemetic, Antipsychotic

Comtan, Comtess	Entacapone	Antiparkinson Agent-Catechol O-Methyltransferase (COMT) Inhibitor
Comvax	Influenza B and Hepatitis B Vaccine	Vaccine
Conceptrol Disposable Contraceptive	Nonoxynol 9 Vaginal Gel	Spermicide Contraceptive
Condylox, Condyline	Podofilox	Antiviral
Conjugated Estrogens with Methyltestosterone	Premarin w/ Methyltestosterone	Androgen/Estrogen Combination
Conray 30	Iothalamate Meglumine 30%	Diagnostic Aid
Conray 325	Iothalamate Sodium 54.3%	Diagnostic Aid
Conray 400	Iothalamate Sodium 66.8%	Diagnostic Aid
Conray 43	Iothalamate Meglumine 43%	Diagnostic Aid
Conray 60	Iothalamate Meglumine 60%	Diagnostic Aid
ConXn	Recombinant Human Relaxin	Tx of scleroderma
Copaxone	Glatiramer Acetate (Copolymer-1)	Biologic Response Modifer
Cordarone, Pacerone	Amiodarone HCl	Antiarrythmic, Group III Antiarrhythmic

Cordox	Fructose Diphosphate (Fructose-1, 6-Diphosphate)	Tx of sickle cell disease
Cordran, Cordran SP	Flurandrenolide	Antiinflammatory
Coreg	Carvediol	Antihypertensive, ß-Adrenergic Blocker
Corgard	Nadolol	ß-Adrenergic Blocker, Antihypertensive, Antianginal
Corlopam	Fenoldopam Mesylate	Antihypertensive, vasodilator
Cortef Oral Suspension	Hydrocortisone Cypionate	Corticosteroid Glucocorticoid
Cortef, Hydrocortone	Hydrocortisone Oral	Glucocorticoid
Cortenema, Colocort	Hydrocortisone Enema	Glucocorticoid Retention Enema
Cortisporin	Hydrocortisone, Neomycin, Polymyxin Topical	Steroid/Antibiotic
Cortisporin Ophth.Oint	Hydrocortisone, Neomycin, Polymyxin Ophthalmic Oint.	Ophth. Antibacterial and Antiinflammatory
Cortisporin Ophth.Susp	Hydrocortisone, Neomycin, Polymyxin Ophthalmic Susp.	Ophth. Antibacterial and Antiinflammatory

Cortisporin Otic, Pediotic	Hydrocortisone, Neomycin, Polymyxin Otic	Tx of otitis externa
Cortisporin TC	Hydrocortisone, Neomycin, Thonzium, Colistin otic	Tx of otitis externa
Cortone	Cortisone Acetate	Glucocorticoid
Cortrosyn, Synacthen	Cosyntropin	Diagnostic Agent
Corvert	Ibutilide Fumarate	Antiarrhythmic
Corzide	Bendroflumethiazide & Nadolol	Antihypertensive
Cosmegen	Actinomycin-D	Antineoplastic
Cosmegen	Dactinomycin	Antineoplastic
Cosopt	Dorzolamide & Timolol	Antiglaucoma
Cotazym, Viokase, Creon, Ilozyme, Lipram, Pancrease, Ultras, Ku-Zyme, Protilase	Pancrelipase	Digestive Enzymes
Coumadin, (Compound-42)	Warfarin	Anticoagulant
Coviracil, FTC	Emtricitabine	Antiviral
Cozaar	Losartan Potassium	Antihypertensive
Crestor, ZD4522	Rosuvastatin	Tx of hyperlipidemia
Crixivan	Indinavir	Antiviral
CroFab	Polyvalent crotalide antivenom, ovine Fab	Antivenom for rattlesnake bites

Cromagen Capsules	Hematinic Concentrate with Intrinsic Factor	Hematinic
Cryptaz	Nitazoxanide	Tx of cryptosporidiosis
Crysticillin-AS, Pfizerpen-AS, Wycillin	Penicillin-G Procaine	Antibiotic
Crysticillin-AS, Pfizerpen-AS, Wycillin	Procaine Penicillin	Antibiotic
Crystodigin	Digitoxin	Ionotropic Agent
Cuprimine, Depen	Penicillamine	Chelating Agent (Copper Toxicity)
Curosurf	Poractant alfa	Pulmonary Surfactant
Cutivate	Fluticasone Propionate Topical	Antiinflammatory
Cyanocobolamin	Vitamin B12	Vitamin
Cyclan, Cyclospasmol	Cyclandelate	Peripheral Vasodilator
Cyclocort	Amcinonide	Topical Corticosteroid
Cyclogyl, Pentolair, AK-Pentolate	Cyclopentolate	Mydriatic, Cycloplegic
Cyclospire	Liposomal Cyclosporin-A	Anti-Rejection
Cyklokapron	Tranexamic Acid	Systemic Hemostatic
Cylert	Pemoline	CNS Stimulant
Cystadane	Betaine	Miscellaneous Agent
Cystagon	Cysteamine Bitartrate	Urinary Tract

Cysto Conray (not intended for intravascular admin)	Iothalamate Meglumine 43%	Diagnostic Aid
Cystografin Dilute (not for IV admin.)	Diatrizoate Meglumine 18%	Diagnostic Aid
Cystografin, Hypaque-Cysto, Remo-M-30, Urovist Cysto (not for IV admin)	Diatrizoate Meglumine 30%	Diagnostic Aid
Cytadren	Aminoglutethimide	Adrenal steroid inhibitor
CytoGam	Cytomegalovirus immune globulin IV (CMV-IGIV)	For CMV disease
Cytomel, Triostat	Liothyronine Sodium, (T3)	Thyroid Replacement
Cytosar-U, Cytosine Arabinoside, ARA-C	Cytarabine	Antineoplastic
Cytotec, PGE1	Misoprostol	Prostaglandin
Cytovene I.V.	Ganciclovir Sodium	Antiviral
Cytovene, DHPG	Ganciclovir	Antiviral
Cytoxan, Neosar	Cyclophosphamide	Antineoplastic
Dalcipran	Dalcipran	Antidepressant
Dalgan	Dezocine	Opioid Analgesic
Dalmane Somnol, Som Pam	Flurazepam	Sedative, Hypnotic
Danocrine	Danazol	Gonadotropin

		Inhibitor
Dantrium	Dantrolene Sodium	Skeletal Muscle Relaxant
Daranide	Dichlorphenamide	Antiglaucoma agent
Daraprim	Pyrimethamine	Antimalarial
Daricon	Oxyphencyclimine HCl	GI Anticholinergic, Antispasmodic
Darvocet-N 50, Darvocet-N 100, Propacet	Propoxyphene Napsylate and Acetaminophen	Analgesic, Opioid Agonist
Darvon Compound-65	Propoxyphene HCl, Aspirin and Caffeine	Analgesic, Opioid Agonist
Darvon, Dolene	Propoxyphene HCl (Dextroproxyphene)	Analgesic, Opiate agonist
Darvon-N	Propoxyphene Napsylate (Dextroproxyphene)	Analgesic, Opioid Agonist
DaunoXome, Cerubidine	Daunorubicin Citrate Liposome Injection	Antineoplastic
Daypro	Oxaprozin	Analgesic, Antiinflammatory
DBI	Phenformin	Biguanide Hypoglycemic Agent
DDAVP, Stimate, Octostim	Desmopressin Acetate	Posterior Pituitary Hormone, Anti-Enuretic Agent

Debrisan	Dextranomer	For cleaning wet ulcers and wounds
Debrox, Auro	Carbamide Peroxide (Urea Peroxide) Otic Solution	Cerumenolytic, Antiinfective
Decabid	Indecainide HCl	Antiarrhythmic
Decadron Phosphate, Dalalone, Decaject, Dexasone, Dexone, Solurex, Cortastat, Hexadrol Phosphate	Dexamethasone Sodium Phosphate	Corticosteroid, Glucocorticoid
Decadron w/Xylocaine	Dexamethasone Sodium Phosphate and Lidocaine	Injectable Steroid and Local Anesthetic Combination
Decadron, Hexadrol, Dexameth, Dexone, Dexamethasone Intensol, Dexasone	Dexamethasone	Corticosteroid, Glucocorticoid
Decadron-LA, Dalalone L.A., Decaject-L.A., Dexene LA, Solurex LA, Dalaone D.P.	Dexamethasone Acetate	Corticosteroid, Glucocorticoid
Decholin, Cholan-	Dehydrocholic	Hydrocholeretic

HMB	Acid	
Declomycin	Demeclocycline	Antibiotic
DEHOP	Diethylhomospermine	Polyamine Analogue, Antidiarrheal Agent
Delaprem	Hexoprenaline Sulfate	Tocolytic Agent
Delatestryl, Andro L.A., Andropository, Durathate, Everone	Testosterone Enthanate	Androgen, long acting
Delestrogen, Estra-L, Valergen, Dioval XX, Gynogen LA	Estradiol Valerate	Hormone
Delfen Contraceptive, Because, Emko, Emko Pre-Fil	Nonoxynol 9 Vaginal Foam	Spermicide Contraceptive
Demadex	Torsemide	Diuretic
Demerol, Pethidine	MeperidineHCl	Narcotic Analgesic
Demser	Metyrosine	Antihypertensive
Denavir	Penciclovir	Antiviral
Depacon	Valproate Sodium	Anticonvulsant
Depakene, Deproic, Epiject, Epival	Valproic Acid	Anticonvulsant
Depakote	Divalproex Sodium	Anticonvulsant
Depakote-ER	Divalproex Extended Release	Prevention of Migraines in Adults
DepoCyt	Cytarabine Liposome	Antineoplastic

Depo-Estradiol Cypionate, DepoGen, depGynogen	Estradiol Cypionate in Oil	Estrogen
Depo-Medrol, Adlone, depMedalone, Depoject, Depopred, D-Med, Medralone, M-Prednisol	Methylprednisolone Acetate	Glucocorticoid
DepoMorphine	Morphine sustained release injection	Analgesic
Depo-Provera	Medroxyprogesterone Acetate Injection	Antineoplastic, Inject. Contraceptive
Depo-Testadiol, Depotestogen, Duo-Cyp, Duratestrin, DepAndroglyn, Test-Estro Cypionate	Estradiol Cypionate and Testosterone Cypionate	Estrogen & Androgen Combination
Depo-Testosterone, depAndro, Depotest, Duratest	Testosterone Cypionate	Androgen, long acting
Deprol	Benactyzine HCl & Meprobamate	Antianxiety, Antidepressant
Dermatop	Prednicarbate	Antiinflammatory
Dermex II	Zinc Oxinate	Tx of actinic keratosis

Desenex, Cruex, Decyclenes, Fungoid AC, Caldesene, PediDri, Protectol, FungiNail, Undoguent, PediPro, Merlenate	Undecylenic Acid	Antifungal
Desferal Mesylate	Deferoxamine Mesylate	Chelate Iron
Desoxyn, Methadrine	Methamphetamine HCl	CNS Stimulant, Anorexiant
Desquam, Persa-Gel, Benzac, Clearsil, Acetoxyl	Benzoyl Peroxide	Acne Product
Desyrel	Trazodone	Antidepressant
Detrol	Tolterodine	Antimuscarinic, for Bladder Spasms
Detrol LA	Tolterodine Tartrate Extended Release	Anticholinergic
Dexedrine, DextroStat, Ferndex	Dextroamphetamine Sulfate	CNS Stimulant
DHC Plus Capsules	Acetaminophen, Caffeine and Dihydrocodeine Bitartrate	Analgesic
DHE 45 (inj), Migranal (nasal spray)	Dihydroergotamine Mesylate	Sympatholytic Agent for Migraines
DHEA, Alsera	Dehydroepiandrosterone sulfate	Accelerate re-epithelialization

	sodium	
DHT, Hytakerol	Dihydrotachysterol	Vitamin D Analog
DiaBeta, Glynase, Micronase, Euglucon	Glyburide (Glibenclamide)	Antidiabetic
Diabinese	Chlorpropamide	Antidiabetic
Dialose Plus, Peri-Colace, Geri-Care	Docusate Potassium with Casanthranol	Laxative, stool softener
Diamox	Acetazolamide	Diuretic, Anticonvulsant, Antiglaucoma
Diapid	Lypressin (8-Lysine Vasopressin)	For Diabetes Insipidus
Diatrizoate Meglumine	Diatrizoate Meglumine 76%	Diagnostic Aid
Dibenzyline	Phenoxybenzaine HCl	Antihypertensive
Diclectin, Bendectin	Doxylamine succinate and pyridoxine HCl	For Nausea/Vomiting associated with pregnancy
Dicumarol	Dicumarol	Anticoagulant
Didrex	Benzphetamine	Anorexiant
Didronel	Etidronate Disodium	Bisphosphonate
Differin	Adapalene	Dermatologic-Acne
Diflucan	Fluconazole	Antifungal
Digibind, Digidote	Digoxin Immune Fab	Antidote for Digoxin Overdose

Dilantin	Phenytoin Sodium, Extended	Anticonvulsant
Dilantin, Phenytoin Prompt	Phenytoin Sodium, Prompt	Anticonvulsant
Dilantin, Phenytoin, Diphen, Tremytoine	Diphenylhydantoin	Anticonvulsant
Dilaudid Cough Syrup	Hydromorphone and Guaifenesin	Antitussive
Dilaudid, Dilaudid-HP, Dilaudid-5	Hydromorphone HCl	Narcotic
Dilor-G, Dyflex-G, Dyline G.G., Lufyllin G.G.	Dyphylline and Guaifenesin	Bronchodilator, Mucolytic
Dimetane	Brompheniramine Maleate	Antihistamine
Dimetapp	Brompheniramine Maleate & Phenylpropanolamine HCl	Antihistamine, Decongestant
Dionosil Oily (not intended for intravascular admin)	Propyliodione 60% in Peanut Oil	Diagnostic Aid
Diovan	Valsartan	Antihypertensive
Diovan-HCT	Valsartan/HCTZ	Antihypertensive
Dipentum	Olsalazine Sodium	Antiinflammatory
Diprivan	Propofol	General Anesthetic
Diprolene	Augmented Betamethasone Dipropionate	Top. Steroid

Diprosone, Maxivate	Betamethasone Dipropionate	Topical Anti-inflammatory
Dip-Tet, Tet-Dip	Diptheria-Tetanus Toxoid	Immunization
Dirame, Bay-4503	Propiram Fumarate	Opioid Analgesic
Disalcid, Salflex	Salsalate	Antiinflammatory
Ditropan	Oxybutynin	Antimuscarinic, for Bladder Spasms
Ditropan-XL	Oxybutynin Extended Release Tables	Antimuscarinic, for Bladder Spasms
Diucardin, Salurn	Hydroflumethiazide	Diuretic, Antihypertensive
Diuril	Chlorothiazide	Diuretic
Diutensen-R	Reserpine and methyclothiazide	Antihypertensive
DMP-450	Mozenavir	Antiretroviral Agent
Dobutrex	Dobutamine HCl	Sympathomimetic Vasopressor
Dolobid	Diflunisal	Analgesic, Antiinflammatory
Dolophene, Methadose	Methadone HCl	Narcotic Analgesic
Dolorac	Capsaicin	Topical Analgesic
Domeboro Otic, VoSol Otic	Acetic Acid Otic	Otic Antiinfective
Donnagel	Kaolin, Pectin and Belladonna	Antidiarrhea Agent
Donnagel-PG	Kaolin, Pectin and Opium	Antidiarrhea Agent

Donnatal Extentabs	Belladonna Alkaloids & Phenobarbital Extended Release	GI-Antichohinergic, Antispasmotic
Donnatal, Hyosophen, Antispasmotic, Susano, Belhacane Elixirs	Belladonna Alkaloids & Phenobarbital Liquid	GI-Antichohinergic, Antispasmotic
Donnatal, Hyosophen, Spasmolin, Barbidonna	Belladonna Alkaloids & Phenobarbital	GI-Antichohinergic, Antispasmotic
Donnazyme, Pancrezyme, Creon, Digespepsin	Pancreatin	Digestive Enzymes
Dopar, Larodopa	Levodopa	Antiparkinson Agent
Dopascan	I-123 Radiolabeled Tropane Derivative	Dx of Parkinson's Disease
Dopram	Doxapram	Respiratory Stimulant, Cerebral Stimulant
Doral	Quazepam	Sedative, Hypnotic
Dostinex	Cabergoline	Antihyperprolacinemic
Dovonex	Calcipotriene Topical	Tx of plaque psoriasis
Doxidan-changed formula	Docusate Calcium with Phenolphthalein	Laxative, stool softener
Doxil, Evacet	Doxorubicin Liposome Injection	Antineoplastic

DPT	Diptheria, Tetanus, Pertussis	Immunization
Dramamine, Gravol, Travel Tabs	Dimenhydrinate	Antivertigo, Antiemetic
DTIC-Dome	Dacarbazine	Antineoplastic
Dulcolax, Correctol, Feen-a-Mint	Bisacodyl	Laxitive
DuoDerm, DuoDerm CGF, DuoDerm Extra Thin	Flexible Hydroactive Dressings and Granules	Protective Dressing
DuoNeb	Ipratropium and Albuterol Inhalent Sol.	Bronchodilator Anticholinergic combination
Durabolin, Hybolin	Nandrolone Phenpropionate	Anabolic Steroid
Duraclon	Clonidine Inj.	Non-Opiod Analgesic
Duragesic	Fentanyl Patch	Narcotic Analgesic
Duranest	Etidocaine HCl	Local Anesthetic
Duranest with Epinephrine	Etidocaine with Epinephrine	Local Anesthetic
DuraPac	Fluoxetine HCl Extended Release	Antidepressant, SSRI
Duricef, Ultricef	Cefadroxil	Antibiotic
Dycill, Dynapen, Pathocil	Dicloxacillin Sodium	Antibiotic
Dymelor	Acetohexamide	Antidiabetic
Dynabac	Dirithromycin	Antibiotic

DynaCirc, DynaCirc-CR	Isradipine	Calcium Channel Blocker, Antihypertensive
Dyrenium	Triamterene	Diuretic
Ecotrin	Aspirin E.C.	Analgesic, Antipyretic
Ecotrin	Enteric Coated Aspirin	Analgesic, Antipruitic, Antiplatelet
Ecotrin, Empirin, ASA, Bayer, Halfprin, Entrophen, ZORprin, Asaphen	Aspirin	Analgesic, Antipyretic, Antiplatelet Agent
Ecovia	Remacemide HCl	Tx of Huntington's Chorea and for Epilepsy
Edecrin	Ethacrynic Acid	Diuretic
Edronax, Vestra	Reboxetine	Antidepressant
EES, EryPed	Erythromycin Ethylsuccinate	Antibiotic
Effexor	Venlafaxine	Antidepressant
Eflone, Flarex	Fluorometholone Acetate	Anti-Inflammatory
Efudex, Fluoroplex, 5FU, Carac (0.5%)	Fluorouracil Topical	Antineoplastic
Elavil, Endep, Vanatrip, Levate	Amitriptyline HCl	Antidepressant, TCA
Eldepryl Patch	Selegiline Transdermal	MAOI Antidepressant, Tx of Aizheimer's
Eldepryl, Carbex, Deprenyl,	Selegiline HCl	MAOI Antidepressant

Deprenil, Selpak		
Eldisine, DAVA	Vindesine Sulfate	Antineoplastic
Eldopaque, Eldoquin, Esoterica, Porcelana, Solaquin	Hydroquinone Cm. 2%	Skin Bleach
Elimite, Acticin, Nix, Kwellada-P	Permethrin	Scabicide, pediculicide
Elixophyllin, TheoDur, SloPhyllin, SloBid, Constant-T, Aerolate	Theophylline	Bronchodilater
Ellence, Farmorubicin	Epirubicin	Antineoplastic
Elmiron	Pentosan Polysulfate Sodium	Urinary Analgesic, Tx of interstitial cystitis
Elocon	Mometasone Topical	Antiinflammitory
Eloxatin	Oxaliplatin	Antineoplastic
Elspar, Oncaspar	Asparaginase (Pegaspargase)	Antineoplastic
Emadine	Emedastine	Antiallergic, ophthalmic antihistamine
Emcyt	Estramusine	Antineoplastic
Emete-Con	Benzquinamide HCl	Antiemetic

Emetrol, Nausetrol	Phosphated Carbohydrate Solution	Antiemetic
Eminase	Anistreplase, (APSAC) Anisoylated PSAC	Thrombolytic
Emitasol	Metoclopramide Intranasal Spray	Tx of acute & delayed emesis of chemotherapy
EMLA	Lidocaine and Prilocaine	Local Anesthetic, Topical
Empirin with Codeine	Aspirin with Codeine	Analgesic, Narcotic
E-Mycin, ERYC, E-Base Ery-Tab, Ilotycin, PCE	Erythromycin Base	Antibiotic
Enable	Tenidap	Antiinflammatory
Enbrel	Etanercept	Treatment of rheumatoid arthritis
Encare, Conceptrol Contraceptive inserts, Semicid	Nonoxynol 9 Vaginal	Spermicide Contraceptive
Enduronyl, Enduronyl Forte	Methyclothiazide and Deserpidine	Antihypertensive
Engerix-B, Recombivax-HB, Heptavax	Hepatitis-B Vaccine	Vaccine
Enkaid	Encainide	Group I-C Antiarrhythmic
Enlon Plus	Edrophonium and Atropine	Muscle Stimulant

Enlon, Reversol, Tensilon	Edrophonium Chloride	Cholinomimetic, Cholinergic Muscle Stimulant, Diagnostic for Myasthenia Gravis
Entex-LA	Guaifenesin Phenylpropanolamine	Mucolytic, Decongestant
Entex-LA, Guaitex-LA	Phenylpropanolamine HCl & Guaifenesin	Decongestant and Expectorant
Entex-PSE, Congestac	Guaifenesin and Pseudoephridine	Mucolytic decongestant combo.
Entocort CR	Budesonide oral	Steroid
Ephedrine	Ephedrine Sulfate	Bronchodilator
Epifrin	Epinephrine HCl Ophth.	Antiglaucoma Agent
Epinal	Epinephrine Borate	Antiglaucoma agent
EpiPen	Epinephrine HCl Auto-injector	Tx of allergic Rx
Epivir, 3-TC, Heptovir, Epivir-HB	Lamivudine	Antiviral
Epogen, Procrit, EPO	Epoetin Alfa	Stimuate red blood cell production
Epsom Salt	Magnesium Sulfate	Saline Laxative
Equagesic	Meprobamate & Aspirin	Analgesic, Anxiolytic
Ergamisol	Levamisole HCl	Immunomodulator
Ergocalciferol	Vitamin D2	Vitamin
Ergomar, Ergostat	Ergotamine Tartrate	Antimigraine

Ergotrate Maleate	Ergonovine Maleate	Oxytocic
Erwinase, (Porton Asparaginase)	Erwinia L-Asparaginase	Antineoplastic
Erythrocin IV	Erythromycin Lactobionate	Antibiotic
Erythrocin Stearate, Eramycin	Erythromycin Stearate	Antibiotic
Eserine	Physostigmine	Antiglaucoma
Esoterica Sensitive Skin Formula	Hydroquinone Cm1.5%	Skin Bleach
Estinyl	Ethinyl Estradiol	Hormone
Estrace, Innofen	Estradiol	Hormone
Estraderm , FemPatch, Vivelle, Alora, Climara, Esclim	Estradiol Transdermal	Hormone
Estratab, Menest	Esterified Estrogens	Estrogen
Estratest, Estratest HS	Esterified Estrogens & Methyltestosterone	Estrogen & Androgen Combination
Estring	Estradiol Vaginal Ring	Estrogen
Estrone Aqueous, Kestrone 5, Primestrin, EstraGyn 5	Estrone	Estrogen
Estrostep-21, Estrostep-Fe	Ethinyl Estradiol and Norethindrone 1mg	Contraceptive
ET-743	Ecteinascidin	Anticancer

Ethamolin	Ethanolamine Oleate	Parenteral Sclerosing Agent
Ethaquin, Ethatab, Ethavex-100, Isovex	Ethaverine HCl	Peripheral Vasodilator
Ethezyme, Accuzyme	Papain-Urea Ointment	Debriding Ointment
Ethiodol (not intended for intravascular Admin)	Ethiodized Oil	Diagnostic Aid
Ethmozine	Moricizine HCl	Group I-A Antiarrhythmic
Ethrane	Enflurane	General Anesthetic
Ethyl Chloride	Chloroethane	Local Anesthetic
Ethyol	Amifostine	Cytoprotective agent
Etrafon, Triavil	Amitriptyline, Perphenazine	Antidepressant, Psychotherapeutic
Etrafon, Triavil	Perphenazine & Amitriptyline	Psychotherapeutic Combination
Eulexin, Euflex	Flutamide	Antineoplastic
Eurax, Crotan	Crotamiton	Tx of lice, Scabicide
Euthroid, Thyrolar	Liotrix (1gr = T3/T4 12.5mcg/50 mcg)	Thyroid Replacement
Evacet, Doxil, Caelyx	Doxorobicin, Liposomal	Antineoplastic
Evista	Raloxifene	Antisteoporotic
Evoxac	Cevimeline	Tx of dry mouth with Sjögren's Syndrome

Exanta	Ximelagatran	Oral DirectThrombin Inhibitor
Excedrin Migraine	Acetaminophen, Aspirin & Caffeine	Analgesic/Antipyretic
Exelderm	Sulconazole Nitrate	Antifungal
Exelon	Rivastigmine Tartrate	Alzheimer's Disease
Exna, Aquatag, Hydrex, Proaqua	Benzthiazide	Thiazide Diuretic
Exosurf	Colfosceril Palmitate	Lung Surfactant
Exubera	Insulin, Inhaled	Tx of Diabetes Mellitus
Fabrase, Replagal, CC-Galactosidase	Alpha-galactosidase A	Tx of Fabry Disease
Fabrazyme	Agalsidase ß	Tx of Fabry Disease
Factive	Gemifloxacin Mesylate	3rd Gen Quinolone Antibiotic
Famvir	Famciclovir	Antiviral
Fansidar	Sulfadoxine and Pyrimethamine	Antimalarial
Fareston	Toremifene	Antineoplastic
Faslodex	Fulvestrant	Hormone
Faslodext	ICI182,780	Tx of breast cancer

Fastin, Zantryl, Phentrol, Ionamin, OBY-CAP, Adipex-P, Obenix, Obephen, Obermine, Obestin, Phentamine, Phentride, T-Diet, Zantryl, Obe-Nix, Phentercot, Teramine, OBY-Trim	Phentermine HCl	Anorexiant
Fasturtec	Rasburicase	Prevention and Tx of chemotherapy induced hyperuricemia related to hematologic malignancies
Felbatol	Felbamate	Anticonvulsant
Feldene, Fexicam	Piroxicam	Antiinflammatory, Analgesic
Femara	Letrozole	Antineoplastic
FemBack Caplets	APAP, Salicylamide and Phenyltoloxamine	Analgesic
Femhrt 1/5	Norethindrone Acetate & Ethinyl Estradiol	Hormone Replacement Therapy
Femiron	Ferrous Fumarate	Hematinic
Fentanyl Oralet	Fentanyl Lozenge	Narcotic Analgesic
Fergon	Ferrous Gluconate	Hematinic

Ferrlecit, Iron Gluconate	Sodium Ferric Gluconate Complex	Hematinic
Ferro-Sequels	Ferrous Fumarate with Docusate	Hematinic
Fertinex, Metrodin	Urofollitropin	Ovulation Stimulant
Fe-Tinic 150 Forte	Iron, Folic Acid and Vitamin B-12	Hematinic
FiberCon, Mitrolan, Fiberall, Equalactin	Polycarbophil	Bulk Producing Laxative
Fioricet	Butalbital, Caffeine & Acetaminophen	Sedative analgesic
Fiorinal	Butalbital, Caffeine & Aspirin	Sedative analgesic
Fiorinal with Codeine	Butalbital, Caffeine, Aspirin and Codeine	Narcotic analgesic
Flagyl, Metryl, Metizol, Protostat, Flagyl ER, Trikacide	Metronidazole	Antibiotic
Flaxedil	Gallamine Triethiodide	Nondepolarizing Neuromuscular Blocking Agent
Fleet Enema, Fleet Phospho Soda, Visicol, Diacol	Sodium Phosphates	Laxative
Flesinoxin	Flesinoxan	Antidepressant
Flexeril	Cyclobenzaprine	Skeletal Muscle Relaxant

Flocor	Poloxamer 188	Vasospasm, Sickle cell crisis, severe burns
Flocor	Polyxamer 188	Tx of sickle cell crisis
Flolan, PGl2, PGX, Epoprostenol	Prostacyclin	Antihypertensive
Flolan, PGl2, PGX, Prostaglandin I2, Prostacyclin	Epoprostenol	Antihypertensive
Flomax	Tamsulosin	BPH
Flonase, Flovent, Flovent Diskus	Fluticasone Propionate	Antiinflammitory
Florinef	Fludrocortisone Acetate	Steroid
Florone, Maxiflor, Psorcon	Diflorasone Diacetate	Corticosteroid
Floropryl	Isoflurophate	Antiglaucoma
Floxin	Ofloxacin Oral	Antibiotic
Floxin Otic	Ofloxacin ottc	Tx of otitis externa
Fludara	Fludarabine Phosphate	Antineoplastic
Flumadine	Rimantadine HCl	Antiviral, Influenza A
FluMist Vaccine	Influenza Vaccine nasal spray	Vaccine
Fluorescite, Fluor-I-Strip	Fluorescein Sodium	Misc. EENT Diagnostic
Fluori-Methane	Chlorofluoromethane	Local Anesthetic
Fluothane	Halothane	General Anesthetic

Fluress	Fluresceine and Benoxinate	Dignostic Aget
Fluzone, Fluvirin, FluShield, Fluogen, Fluviral, Vaxigrip	Influenza Vaccine	Vaccine
FML, FML Forte	Fluorometholone	Anti-Inflammatory
Folex, Rheumatrex, Trexall, MTX	Methotrexate	Antineoplastic, Antipsoriatic, Antirheumatic
Follistim, Gonal-F, r-FSH	Follitropin Beta	Ovulation Stimulant
Foltrin, Contrin, Trinsicon, Ferotrinsic, Livitrinsic-f	Hematinic Concentrate with Intrinsic Factor	Hematinic
Folvite	Folic Acid (Folate, Pteroylglutamic Acid)	Vitamin
Foradil Aerolizer	Formoterol Fumarate	Long acting ß-2 agonist w rapid onset
Forane	Isoflurane	General Anesthetic
Fortaz, Tazidime, Tazicef, Pentacef, Ceptaz	Ceftazidime	Antibiotic
Forteo, Parathar	Teriparatide	Parathyroid Hormone
Fortovase	Saquinavir Soft Gelatin Capsules	Antiviral, Protease Inhibitor (PI)
Fosamax	Alendronate Sodium	Bone Resorption Inhibitor, Bisphosphonate

Foscan	Temoporfin	Antineoplastic
Foscavir	Foscarnet Sodium	Antiviral
Fragmin	Dalteparin	Anticoagulant
Freedox	Tirilazad	A 21-aminosteroid with distinct antioxidant properties
Frisium	Clobazam	Benzodiazepine
FUDR	Floxuridine	Antineoplastic
Fulvicin-PG, Gris-PEG, Grisactin Ultra, Griseostatin	Griseofulvin Ultramicrosize	Antifungal
Fungizone	Amphotericin B Topical	Antifungal
Fungizone, Amphocin, Fungilin	Amphotericin-B	Antibiotic (Polyene Antifungal)
Furacin	Nitrofurazone	Burn Preparation
Furadantin	Nitrofurantoin	Urinary Antibiotic
Furamide	Diloxanide furoate	Antiinfective
Furoxone	Furazolidone	Antiprotozoal
Gabitril	Tiagabine	Anticonvulsant
Galzin	Zinc acetate	Tx of Wilson's disease
Gamastan, Gammar	Gamma Globulin IM	Serum
Gamimune, Gammagard, Gammar-IV, IVIG, Sandoglobulin, Panglobulin, Polygam, Venoglobulin	Immune globulin IV	Serum

Gamimune-N, Gammar, IMIG	Immune Globulin IM	Serum
Ganite	Gallium Nitrate	For cancer related hypercalcemia
Gantanol	Sulfamethoxazole	Antiinfective Agent
Gantrisin	Sulfisoxazole	Antibiotic
Gantrisin Ophth. Sol.	Sulfisoxazole Diolamine	Antibiotic
Garamycin Topical, G-Myticin	Gentamicin Topical	Topical Antibiotic
Garamycin, Janamicin, Cidomycin	Gentamicin Parenteral	Antibiotic
Gastrimmune	Anti-Gastrin Vaccine	Tx of a variety of GI cancers and other GI diseases
Gastrimmune	Gastrointestinal Cancer Vaccine	Tx of gastric cancer
Gastrografin, MD-Gastroview	Diatrizoate Meglumine 66% and Diatrizoate Sodium 10%	Diagnostic Aid
Gastrozepine	Pirenzepine HCl	Tricyclic benzodiazepine
Gax-X, Mylicon, Phazyme, Mylanta Gas, Gas Relief, Maalox Anti-Gas Genasyme, Baby Gas Relief	Simethicone	Antiflatulant

Gelpirin	APAP, Aspirin, and Caffeine	Analgesic
Gemzar	Gemcitabine HCl	Antineoplastic Agent
Genoptic, Garamycin Ophthalmic, Alcomicin	Gentamicin Ophthalmic	EENT Antibiotic
Geocillin	Carbenicillin Indanyl Sodium	Antibiotic
Geodon, Zeldox	Ziprasidone	Antipsychotic
Geopen	Carbenicillin Disodium	Antibiotic
Gleevec (STI-571) (Glivec)	Imatinib Mesylate	Tx of chronic myelogenous leukemia
GlucaGen	Glucagon (rDNA origin)	Tx of severe hypoglycemic Rxns
Glucagon, GlucaGen (rDNA origin glucagon)	Glucagon	Tx of severe hypoglycemic Rxns
Glucophage, Glucophage XR, Glycon	Metformin	Oral Hypoglycemic (biguanide class)
Glucotrol, Glucotrol-XL	Glipizide	Antidiabetic
Glucovance	Glyburide & Metformin	Antidiabetic
Glutofac-MX, Glutofac	Multimineral Supplement with Iron	Dietary Supplement
Glutofac-ZX	Multimineral Supplement	Dietary Supplement

Glutose, B-D Glucose, Insta-Glucose	Dextrose	Tx of hypoglycemia
Glycine for Irrigation	Aminoacetic Acid Solution for Irrigation	For bladder irrigation
Gly-Oxide	Carbamide .(Urea) Peroxide Solution	local anti-infective
Glypressin	Terlipressin	Bleeding esophageal varices
Glyquin, Nuguin HP, Eldopague-Forte, Solaguin Forte, Melquin HP, Melpaque HP, Alustra	Hydroquinone Cm. 4%	Skin Bleach
Glyset	Miglitol	Antidiabetic
GMK	Melanoma Vaccine	Vaccine for malignant melanoma
Go-Lytely, NuLytely, Colyte, Colavage, Klean-Prep, Lyteprep	Polyethylene Glycol 3350 with electrelytes	Laxative
Gonal-F	Follitropin Alfa	Ovulation Stimulant
Goody's Extra Strength Headache Powders	APAP, Aspirin and Caffeine	Analgesic
Granulex	Balsam of Peru/Trypsin Spray	Topical Protectant

Grifulvin V, Grisactin, Fulvicin-UF, Fulcin, Grisovin, Grisovin FP	Griseofulvin Microsize	Antifungal
Guanidine HCl	Guanidine HCl	Cholinergic Muscle Stimulant
Guanidine HCl	Guanidine HCl	Cholinergic muscle stimulant
Gylgrin	Monolaurin	Tx of congenital primary ichthyosis
Gynazole-1,Femstat-3	Butoconazole Nitrate	Topical Antifungal
H.P. Acthar Gel, ACTH-80, H.P. Acthar Gel	Corticotropin Repository Injection	Pituitory Hormone
Habitrol, Nicoderm, Clear Nicoderm, Prostep	Nicotine Transdermal	Smoking Deterrent
Halcion	Triazolam	Anxiolytic, sedative, hypnotic
Haldol	Haloperidol Lactate	Antipsychotic
Haldol Decanoate	Haloperidol Decanoate	Antipsychotic
Haldol, Peridol	Haloperidol	Antipsychotic
Halfan	Halofantrine	Antimalarial
Halog	Halcinonide	Antiinflammatory
Halotestin	Fluoxymesterone	Hormone
Halotex	Haloprogin	Antifungal
Havrix, Vaqta	Hepatitis-A Vaccine	Vaccine

Healon, Amvisc, Duovisc, Hyalgan, Provisc, Synvisc, Viscoat, Vitrax	Sodium Hyaluronate	Ophthalmic Agent, Musculoskeletal Agent
Hectorol	Doxercalciferol	Vitamin D Analog
Helixate FS, Kogenate FS	Factor VIII, Recomibinant	Tx of hemophilia A
Hemabate, (Prostin-15mF2alpha)	Carboprost Tromethamine	Abortifacient, Oxytocic
Hemex	Hemin and zinc mesoporphyrin	Tx of porphyric syndromes
Herceptin	Trastuzumab	Metastatic Breast Cancer
Herplex, Stoxil, Dendrid	Idoxuridine	Antiviral
Hespan, Hextend	Hetastarch	Plasma Volume Expander
Hetrazan	Diethylcarbamazine Citrate	Anthelminic
Hexabrix	Ioxaglate Meglumine 39.3% and Ioxaglate Sodium 19.6%	Diagnostic Aid
Hexalen, HMM hexamethylmelamine,	Altretamine	Antineoplastic
Hibiclens	Chlorhexidine Gluconate Cleanser	Topical Antiinfective
Hiprex, Urex	Methenamine Hippurate	Urinary Anti-infective
Hismanal	Astemizole	Antihistimine

Hivid, ddC	Zalcitabine	Antiviral
HIVIG	HIV Immune Globulin	Tx of AIDS
HMS	Medrysone Ophthalmic	Antiinflammatory
Humabid, Robitussin, Glycerol Guaiacolate, GG-Cen, Fenesin, Organidin NR, Phanasin, Breonesin, Muco-Fen	Guaifenesin	Mucolytic
Humalog	Insulin Lispro	Hormone
Humatin, Gabbromicina, Paromomycin	Aminosidine	Gabbromicina-Tx of TB (M.avium complex) Paromomycin-Tx of visceral leishmaniasis
Humorsol	Demecarium Bromide	Antiglaucoma
Humulin 50/50	Insulin NPH/Regular 50:50 Human	Hormone
Humulin 70/30	Insulin NPH/Regular 70%:30%, Human	Hormone
Humulin-N, Novolin-N	Insulin NPH Human	Hormone
Humulin-R, Novolin-R	Insulin Regular, Human	Hormone
Hycamtin	Topotecan	Antineoplastic

Hycodan, Hydropane, Tussigon, Hydromet	Hydrocodone and Homatropine	Antitussive
Hycomine	Hydrocodone and Phenylpropanlamine	Antitussive Decongestant
Hycotuss, Entuss, Kwelcof, Codiclear DH	Hydrocodone and Guaifenesin	Antitussive, Expectorant
Hydeltrasol, Pediapred, Orapred, Key-Pred-SP	Prednisolone Sodium Phosphate	Glucocorticoid
Hydeltra-TBA, Prednisol-TBA	Prednisolone Tebutate	Glucocorticoid
Hydergine, Gerimal	Ergoloid Mesylates	Miscellaneous Psychotherapeutic Agent
Hydrea, Droxia, Mylocel	Hydroxyurea	Antineoplastic
Hydrocortisone Acetate	Hydrocortisone Acetate Injection	Corticosteroid Glucocorticoid
Hydrocortone	Hydrocortisone Sodium Phosphate	Corticosteroid Glucocorticoid
HydroDiuril, Esidrex, Oretic, HCTZ, Ezide, Microzide, Hydrocot, Aquazide H	Hydrochlorothiazide	Thiazide Diuretic
Hydromox	Quinethazone	Diuretic

Hydropres	Hydrochlorothiazide and Reserpine	Antihypertensive
Hygroton, Thalitone	Chlorthalidone	Diuretic, Antihypertensive
Hylorel	Guanadrel Sulfate	Antihypertensive
Hylutin	Hydroxyprogesterone Caproate	Progestin
Hypaque Meglumine 30%, Reno-M-Dip, Urovist Meglumine	Diatrizoate Meglumine 30%	Diagnostic Aid
Hypaque Sodium	Diatrizoate Sodium	Diagnostic Aid
Hypaque Sodium 20% (not for intravascular admin)	Diatrizoate Sodium 20%	Diagnostic Aid
Hypaque Sodium 255	Diatrizoate Socium 25%	Diagnostic Aid
Hypaque sodium 50%, Urovist Sodium 300	Diatrizoate sodium 50%l	Diagnostic Aid
Hypaque Solution	Diatrizoate Sodium 41.66%	Diagnostic Aid
Hypaque-M 75%	Diatrizoate Meglumine 50% and Diatrizoate Sodium 25%	Diagnostic Aid
Hypaque-M 90%	Diatrizoate Meglumine 60% and Diatrizoate Sodium 30%	Diagnostic Aid

Hyperstat	Diazoxide Injection	Antihypertensive
Hyper-Tet, Baytet	Tetanus Immune Globulin (TIG)	Serum
Hytrin	Terazosin	Antihypertenive also treatment of BPH
Hyzaar	Losartan Potassium & Hydrochlorothiazide	Antihypertensive
Ichthammol, Ichthyol	Ichthammol Ointment	Relief of minor skin irritations
Idamycin	Idarubicin HCl	Antineoplastic
Ifex	Ifosfamide	Antineoplastic
IgE 025A	Anti-IgE	Tx of allergic rhinitis
Ilopan	Dexpanthenol	Post-Op to prevent ileus (prophylaxis)
Ilopan-Choline	Dexpanthenol and Choline Bitartrate	Tx of Flatulence
Ilosone	Erythromycin Estolate	Antibiotic
Ilotycin Gluceptate	Erythromycin Gluceptate	Antibiotic
Ilotycin, AK Mycin	Erythromycin Ophth. Oint.	Ophth. Antibacterial
Imdur, ISMO, Monoket	Isosorbide Mononitrate	Nitrate
Imitrex	Sumatriptan Succinate	Agent for Migraine
Immunol	Complexed prostate specific antigen (cPSA) test	For detection of prostate cancer

Imodium, Imodium-AD, Loperacap	Loperamide HCl	Antidiarrheal
Imogam, BayRab	Rabies Immune Globulin, Human	Immunoglobulin
Imuran	Azathioprine	Immunosuppressant
Imuthiol	Diethyldithiocarbo mate	Tx of AIDS
Inapsine	Droperidol	Antianxiety, Antiemetic
Inderal, Betachron-ER	Propranolol HCl	ß-Adrenergic Blocker, Antihypertensive, Group II Antiarrhythmic
Inderide, Inderide-LA	Propranolol HCl and Hydrochlorothiazid e	Antihypertensive
Indocin I.V.	Indomethacin Sodium Trihydrate	Closure of patents ductus arteriosus in neonates
Indocin, Indocin-SR, Indotec, Indocid	Indomethacin	Anti-inflammatory
InFed, DexFerrum, Dexiron, Infufer	Iron Dextran	Hematinic, Iron Suppliment
Infergen, Consensus Interferon (CIFN)	Interferon Alfacon-1	Antiviral
Inhibace	Cilazapril	Tx of hypertension and CHF

Innohep, Logiparin	Tinzaparin sodium	Anticoagulant
Innovar	Fentanyl and Droperidol	Opiate and Anxiolytic Combination
Inocor	Inamrinone (Amrinone) Lactate	Inotropic
INOmax	Nitric Oxide for inhalation	Neonatal pulmonary vasodilator
Intal, Nasalcrom, Gastrocrom	Cromolyn Sodium	EENT Misc. Drug
Integrilin	Eptifibatide	Antiplatelet
Intrachol	Choline Chloride	Choline deficiency associated with long term parenteral nutrition
IntraDose Injectable Gel	Cisplatin and Epinephrine	Antineoplastic
IntraSite	Graft T Starch Copolymer Hydrogel	Protective Dressing
Intron-A	Interferon Alfa-2b	Antineoplastic
Intropin, Dopastat	Dopamine HCl	Sympathomimet, Vasopressor
Inversine	Mecamylamine HCl	Antihypertensive
Investigational	CS-866	Antihypertensive
Investigational	Eperezolid	Antibiotic
Investigational	Xemilofiban	Antiplatelet
Investigational	Montelukast Injection	Antiasthmatic
Invirase	Saquinavir Hard	Antiviral

	Capsules	
Iophen, R-Gen	Iodinated Glycerol	Expectorant
Iopidine	Apraclonidine	Antiglaucoma agent
Ipecac Syrup	Ipecac	Emetic
Ismelin	Guanethidine Monosulfate	Antihypertensive
Ismotic	Isosorbide	Osmotic Diuretic
Isobutyramide Oral Solution	Isobutyramide	Tx of ß-thalassemia and sickle cell disease
Isoprinosine,	Inosine Pranobex, Inosiplex	Immunomodulating Agent
Isopto Atropine	Atroptne	Mydriatic, Cycloplegic
Isopto Carpine, Pilocar, Piostat, Akarpine, Pilopine	Pilocarpine HCl Ophthalmic	Antiglaucoma
Isopto Homatropine	Homatropine HBr	Mydritic, Cycloplegic
Isopto Hyoscine	Scopolamine HBr	Mydriatic, Cycloplegic
Isopto-Carbachol, Miostat, Miostat, Carboptic, Carbostat	Carbachol	Miotic
Isordil, Sorbitrate, ISDN, Dilatrate-SR	Isosorbide Dinitrate	Nitrate
Isovue-128	Iopamidol 26%	Diagnostic Aid
Isovue-200, Isovue-M 200 (for Intrathecal Use Only)	Iopamidol 41%	Diagnostic Aid

Isovue-300, Isovue-M 300 (for Intrathecal Use)	Iopamidol 61%	Diagnostic Aid
Isovue-370	Iopamidol 76%	Diagnostic Aid
Isuprel	Isoproterenol	Vasopressor
JE-Vax	Japanese Encephalitis Vaccine	Vaccine
Kaletra, ABT-378/r	Lopinavir & Ritonavir	Antiviral
Kantrex	Kanamycin Sulfate	Antibiotic
Kaon	Potassium Gluconate	Electrolyte Replacement
Kaopectate, Diarrest, Diasorb, Donnagel, Diatrol, Kaopek, K-Pek, Parapectolin	Kaolin-Pectin (Atipulgite)	Antidiarrhea Agent
Karidium, Luride, Luride Lozi-Tabs, Pediaflor	Sodium Fluoride	Nutritional Product
K-Dur, Kaon-Cl, Klor, Klorvess, K-Tab, Micro-K, Slow-K, Ten-K, Klor-Conl	Potassium Chloride	Electrolyte Replacement
Keflex, Keftab	Cephalexin	Antibiotic
Keflin	Cephalothin	Antibiotic
Kefurox, Zinacef	Cefuroxime	Antibiotic
Kemadrin	Procyclidine HCl	Antiparkinson Agent
Kenacort, Aristocort, Atolone	Triamcinolone	Corticosteroid, Glucocorticoid

Kenalog, Aristocort, Aristocort A, Trimex	Triamcinolone Acetonide Topical	Anti-inflammatory
Kenalog, Aristocort, Tac-3, Tri-Kort, Trilog	Triamcinolone Acetonide Injection	Anti-inflammatory
Keppra	Levetiracetam	Anticonvulsant - Adjunctive Tx for partial-onset seizures in adults w epilepsy.
Kerlone	Betaxolol	ß-Adrenergic Blocker, Antihypertensive
Kestine, Ebastel, Evastel	Ebastine	Antihistamine
Ketalar	Ketamine HCl	General Anesthetic
Ketek, HMR 3647	Telithromycin	Ketolide Antibiotic
Key-Pred, Predalone, Predcor	Prednisolone Aceteate	Glucocorticoid
Kineret, rHuIL-1 Ra	Anakinra	Tx of rheumatoid arthritis
Kinevac	Sincalide	Hormone Peptide
Klonopin, Rivotril, Clonapam	Clonazepam	Anxiolytic, Anticonvulsant
K-Phos	Potassium Acid Phosphate	Urinary Acidifier
K-Phos M.F., K-Phos No.2	Potassium Acid Phosphate & Sodium Acid Phosphate	Urinary Acidifier

K-Phos Neutral	Sodium Phosphate, Potassium Phosphate & Monobasic Sodium Phosphate	Urinary Acidifier
Kristalose	Lactulose for oral solution	Ammonia Detoxicant, Laxative
Kwell, Kildane, Scabene	Lindane	Antiparasitic, Tx of lice, Scabicide
Kytril	Granisetron	Antiemetic
Lac-Hydrin 12%	Ammonium Lactate (Lactic Acid)	Emollient
Lacipal	Lacidipine	Antihypertensive
Lacril, Isopto Tears, Liquifilm Tears, Muro Tears, Hypotears, Neotears, Tearisol	Methylcellulose Drops (Artificial Tears)	Ophth. Lubricant
Lactobin	Lactobin	Tx of AIDS associated diarrhea
Ladotec	Ladotec	Tx of anxiety
Lamictal	Lamotrigine	Anticonvulsant
Lamisil	Terbinafine HCl	Antifungal
Lamisil DermaGel, Lamisil	Terbinafine Topical	Antifungal
Lampit, Bayer 2502	Nifurtimox	Anttinfective
Lamprene	Clofazimine	Leprostatic
Lamstat	Lamifiban	Tx of unstable angina and non-Q-wave MI

Lanoxin, Lanoxicaps, Digitek	Digoxin	Ionotropic Agent
Lantus	Insulin glargine (rDNA origin) injection	Hormone, Tx of Diabetis Mellitus
Largon	Propiomazine HCl	Sedative, Adjunct for Analgesia
Lariam	Mefloquine HCl	Antimalarial
Lasix	Furosemide	Diuretic
Lescol, Lescol XL	Fluvastatin Sodium	Antihyperlipidemic
Leukeran	Chlorambucil	Antineoplastic
Leukine, GM-CSF	Sargramostim	Stimulate WBC Production
Leuprogel	Leuprolide Acetate Gel	Antineoplastic
Leustatin, 2-CDA, Mylinax	Cladribine	Antineoplastic
Leutech	Radiolabeled Monoclonal Imaging Agent	Imaging Agent for diagnosis of equivocal appendicitis
Levaquin	Levofloxacin	Antibiotic
Levatol	Penbutolol Sulfate	ß-Adrenergic Blocker, Antihypertensive
Levo-Dromoran	Levorphanol Tartrate	Narcotic Analgesic
Levophed	Levarterenol	Vasopressor
Levophed	Norepinephrine Bitartrate	Vasopressor
Levsin PB Drops	Hyoscyamine & Phenobarbital	GI-Antichohinergic, Antispasmotic

	Liguid	
Levsin w/Phenobarbital Tabs, Bellacane Tabs	Hyoscyamine & Phenobarbital	GI-Antichohinergic, Antispasmotic
Levsin, Cystospaz, Anaspaz, Levbid, Levsinex, ED-SPAZ, Donnamar, NuLev, A-Spaz/SL, Medispaz, Hyosol, Hyospaz, Spacol, Spasdel, Symax	Hyoscyamine Sulfate	Anticholinergic Antispasmodic
Levulan Kerastick	Aminolevulinic Acid	Nonhyperkeratotic actinic keratoses (precancerous lesions)
Lexxel	Enalapril Maleate with Felodipine-ER	Antihypertensiv e
Librax, Clindex	Chlordiazepoxide &Clindinium Bromide	GI-Anticholinergic, Anxiolytic
Librium, Libritab	Chlordiazepoxide	Anxiolytic
Lidakol, Abreva	Docosanol	Antiviral
Lidex, Lidex-E, Lyderm, Topactin	Fluocinonide	Anti-inflammatory
Lidoderm	Lidocaine Patch	Topical Analgesic, Local Anesthetic (amide)

Limbitrol	Chlordiazepoxide & Amitriptyline	Anxiolytic antidepressant
Lincocin, Lincorex, L-Mycin	Lincomycin	Antibiotic
Lioresal	Baclofen	Skeletal Muscle Relaxant
Lipitor	Atorvastatin	Antihyperlipidemic
Liquaemin, Hepalean, Unfractionated Heparin	Heparin Sodium	Anticoagulant
Lithane, Lithobid, Eskalith, Lithonate	Lithium Carbonate	Antimaniacal
Lithium Citrate Syrup	Lithium Citrate	Antimaniacal
Lithostat	Acetohydroxamic Acid	Urinary Antiinfective, Tx of Nephrolithiasis
Livostin	Levocabastine Ophth.	Anti-Allergy
Livostin	Levocabestine	Antiallergic, ophthalmic antihistamine
Locilex, Cytolex	Pexiganan Acetate Cream	Tx of Infected Diabetic foot ulcers
Locoid	Hydrocortisone Butyrate	Topical Antiinflammatory
Lodine, Lodine-XL, Ultradol	Etodolac	Analgesic, Antiinflammatory
Lodosyn	Carbidopa	Antiparkinson agent
Lomotil	Diphenoxylate HCl with Atropine	Antidiarrheal

	Sulfate	
Loniten	Minoxidil	Antihypertensive
Lopid	Gemfibrozil	Antilipemic Agent
Lopressor, Betaloc	Metoprolol Tartrate	ß-Adrenergic Blocker, Antihypertensive, Antianginal, Post-MI
Lopressor-HCT	Metoprolol and HCTZ	ß-Adrenergic Blocker and diuretic combo, Antihypertensive
Loprox, Penlac	Ciclopirox Olamine	Topical Antifungal
Lorabid	Loracarbef	Antibiotic
Lorelco	Probucol	Antilipemic Agent
Lorothidol, Bitin	Bithionol	Antiinfectiive
Lotemax, Alrex	Loteprednol Etabonate	Antiinflammatory
Lotensin	Benazepril HCl	Antihypertensive
Lotensin-HCTl	Benazepril and HCTZ	Antihypertensive
Lotrel	Amlopidine & Benazepril HCl	Antihypertensive
Lotrimin, Myclex, Femcare, Myccex-G, Mycelex-7, Canestin, Trivagizole 3 Vaginal, Gyne-Lotrimin	Clotrimazole	Topical Antifungal
Lotrisone	Clotrimazole & Betamethasone	Topical Antifungal and Anti-

		Inflammatory
Lotronex	Alosetron	For irritable bowel syndrome (5-HT3 antagonist)Tx of diarrhea predominant IBS in women.
Lovenox	Enoxaparin Sodium	Anticoagulant
Loxitane, Loxapac	Loxapine	Antipsychotic
Lozol, Mycrox	Indapamide	Diuretic
Ludiomil	Maprotiline HCl	Antidepressant
Lufyllin EPG	Dyphylline, Ephedrine, Guaifenesin and Phenobarbital	Bronchodilator Combination
Lufyllin, Dilor, Neothylline	Dyphylline	Bronchodilator
Lumigan	Bimatoprost	Anti-Glaucoma
Luminal, Solfoton	Phenobarbital	Sedative, Anticonvulsant
Lunelle, Cyclofem	Medroxyprogesterone Acetate & Estradiol Cypionate	Contraceptive
Lupron, Viadur, Oaklide, Lupron Depot, DUROS	Leuprolide Acetate	LH-RH Agonist
Lutrepulse	Gonadorelin acetate	Ovulation induction
Luvox	Fluvoxamine	Antidepressant, Tx of OCD, SSRI
Luxiq	Betamethasone Valerate Foam	Toptcal Antiinflammatory

LYMErix	Lyme Disease Vaccine	Vaccine
Lymphazurin 1% (not intended for intravascular admin)	Isosulfan Blue	Diagnostic Aid
Lysodren	Mitotane, o,p'-DDD	Antineoplastic
Maalox Suspension	Aluminum Hydroxide and Magnesium Hydroxide Suspension	Antacid
Macrobid	Nitrofurantoin Macrocrystals & Monohydrate	Urinary Antibiotic
Macrodantin	Nitrofurantoin Macrocrystals	Urinary Antibiotic
Magan, Doan's, Mobidin	Magnesium Salicylate	Salicylate, Analgesic
Magnesium Hydroxide, MOM	Milk of Magnesia	Osmotic Laxitive Antacid
Magnesium Hydroxide, MOM	MOM (Milk of Magnesia)	Osmotic Laxitive Antacid
Magnesium Sulfate	Magnesium Sulfate Injection	Anticonvulsant, Replacement Preparation
Magnevist	Gadopentetate Dimeglumine	Diagnostic Aid
Magonate, Mag-G, Almora, Magtrate	Magnesium Gluconate	Replacement Preparation

Mag-Ox 400, MagOx, Mag-200, Mag-Ox 400, Uro-Mag	Magnesium Oxide	Replacement Preparation
Mag-Tab SR	Magnesium Lactate Dihydrate	Replacement Preparation
Maitec	Gentamicin liposome injection	Tx of disseminated Mycobacterium avium-intracellulare infection
Malarone	Atovaquone/Proguanil	Antimalarial
Maltsupex	Malt Soup Extract	Bulk Laxative
Mandelamine	Methenamine Mandelate	Urinary Anti-infective
Mandol	Cefamandol	Antibiotic
Maolate	Chlorphenesin Carbamate	Muscle Relaxant
Marcaine, Sensorcaine	Bupivicaine HCl	Local Anesthetic
Marezine	Cyclizine	Antiemetic, Antivertigo
Marinol, THC	Dronabinol {delta-9-THC)	Antiemetic, Appetite Stimulant
Marogen	Epoetin Beta	For Anemia associated with end-stage renal disease
Marplan	Isocarboxazid	Antidepressant
Matulane	Procarbazine HCl	Antineoplastic
Mavik	Trandolapril	Antihypertensive
Maxair	Pirbuterol Acetate	Bronchodilator

Maxalt, Maxalt-MLT	Rizatriptan	5-HT Receptor Agonist
Maxamine	Histamine dihydrochloride	Tx metastatic melanoma in combination with cytokine interleukin-2
Maxaquin	Lomefloxacin HCl	Quinolone Antibiotic
Maxicam	Isoxicam	Analgesic, Antiinflammatory
Maxidex	Dexamethasone Ophthalmic	Corticosteroid
Maximum Pain Relief Pamprin Caplets	APAP, Magnesium Salicylate and Pamabrom	Analgesic
Maximum Strength Aqua-Ban	Pamabrom	Diuretic
Maximum Strength Arthriten	APAP, Magnesium Salicylate and Caffeine, Buffered	Analgesic
Maxipime	Cefepime	Antibiotic
MaxiPost	BMS-204352	Neuroprotective
Maxitrol, Dexacidin, Dexasporin, AK-Trol	Dexamethasone, Polymyxin and Neomycin Opthalmic	Opth. antiinfective and antiinflammatory
Maxzide, Dyazide	Triamterene & Hydrochlorothiazide	Diuretic
Maxzide, Dyazide, Maxzide-25 (25/37.5)	Hydrochlorothiazide and Triamterene	Diuretic, Antihypertensive
MBI-226	Bactolysin	Antibacterial

Mebadin	Dehydroemetine	Antiinfective
Mebaral	Mephobarbital	Anticonvulsant
Meclan	Meclocycline Sulfosalicylate	Acne Product
Meclomen	Meclofenamate Sodium	Analgesic, antiinflammatory
Medihaler Ergotamine	Ergotamine MDI	Antimigraine
Medrol	Methylprednisolone	Glucocorticoid
Mefoxin	Cefoxitin	Antibiotic
Megace Suspension	Megestrol Acetate Suspension	Appetite Stimulant
Megace tablets	Megestrol Acetate Tablets	Antineoplastic (tablets only), Progestin
Melagatran	Melagatrone	Hirudin, Thrombin Inhibitor-Anticoagulant
Melanex	Hydroquinone Solution	Skin Bleach
Mellaril	Thioridazine	Antipsychotic
Menomune-A/C/Y/W-135	Meningococcal Polysaccharide Vaccine	Vaccine
Menoplex Tablets	APAP and Phenyltoloxamine	Analgesic
Mentane	Velnacrine	Tx of Alzheimer's
Mentax, Dr. Scholl's Athlete's Foot Cream	Butenafine	Antifungal
Mepergan, Mepergan Fortis	Meperidine HCl & Promethazine	Narcotic Analgesic Combination

303

Mephyton, Aquamephyton	Phytonadione (Vitamin K-1)	Vitamin
Mepron	Atovaquone	Anti-infective, Antiprotazoal
Meridia	Sibutramine	Anorexiant
Merrem I.V.	Meropenem	Antibiotic
Meruvax II	Rubella Virus, Live Attenuated	Vaccine
Mesantoin	Mephenytoin	Anticonvulsant
Mesnex	Mesna	Cytoprotective Agent
Mestinon, Regonol	Pyridostigmine Bromide	Tx of Myasthenia Gravis
Metaret, Antrypol, Bayer 205, Belganyl, Fourneau 309, Cl-1003, Germanin, Moranyl, Naphuride, Naganol	Suramin	Antiprotozoal Agent
Metastron	Strontium-89	Antineoplastic
Methergine	Methylergonovine Maleate	Oxytocic
Meticorten, Orasone, Deltasone, Panasol-S, Prednicen-M, Sterapred, Prednisone Intensol, Liquid Pred, Winpred,	Prednisone	Glucocorticoid

Metreton		
MetroGel	Metronidazole Vaginal	Antiinfective
Metubine Iodide	Metocurine Iodide	Neuromuscular Blocker
Mevacor, (Mevinolin)	Lovastatin	Antihyperlipidemic
Mexitil	Mexiletine HCl	Group I-B Antiarrhythmic
Mezlin	Mezlocillin Sodium	Antibiotic
Miacalcin Nasal Spray	Calcitonin-Salmon Nasal Spray	Paget's Disease, Hypercalcemia, Osteoporosis
Micardis	Telmisartan	Antihypertensive
Micardis HCT	Telmisartan and Hydrochlorothiazide	Tx of hypertension
Micronor, Nor-QD, Norlutin	Norethindrone	Contraceptive
Micturin	Terodiline HCl	Tx of urinary incontinence
Midamor	Amiloride HCl	Diuretic, Antihypertensive

Midrin, Amidrine, Duradrin, I.D.A. Caps, Iso-Acetazone, Midchlor, Migquin, Migratine, Migrazone, Migrex, Mitride	Isometheptene, Acetaminophen, and Dichloralphenazone	Antimigraine
Mifeprex, RU-486	Mifepristone	abortifacient, progesterone inhibitor
Miguard	Frovatriptan	5-HT Receptor Agonist
Milk of Magnesia	Magnesium Hydroxide	Antacid, Saline Laxative
Milontin Kapseals	Phensuximide	Anticonvulsant
Miltown, Equanil	Meprobamate	Antianxiety, sedative
Minipress	Prazosin	Antihypertensive
Minitran, Nitro-Dur, Transderm Nitro, Deponit, Nitro-Derm, Trinipatch, Nitrek	Nitroglycerin Transdermal	Antianginal Agent
Minizide	Prazosin & Polythiazide	Antihyhpertensive
Minocin, Dynacin	Minocycline HCl	Antibiotic
Mintezol	Thiabendazole	Anthelminic
Miochol-E	Acetylcholine Chloride	Antiglaucoma, Miotic
Miradon	Anisindione	Anticoagulant

Miralax	Polyethylene Glycol 3350, NF Powder	Laxative
Mirena IUD	Levonorgestrel Intrauterine System	Implant Contraceptive
Mithracin	Mithramycin, Plicamycin	Antineoplastic
Mithracin	Plicamycin (Mithramycin)	Antineoplastic
Mitolactol	Dibromoducitol	Antineoplastic
Mitrolan, FiberCon, Fiberall, Equalactin	Calcium Polycarbophil	Laxitive orTx diarrhea
Mivacron	Mivacurium Chloride	Muscle Relaxant
MMR	Measles, Mumps, Rubella Vaccine	Vaccine
Moban	Molindone HCl	Antipsychotic
Mobic	Meloxicam	Antiinflammatory, Analgesic
Moctanin	Monoctanoin	Disselution of cholesterol gallstones retained in the common bile duct
Modane, Alophen, Feen-a-mint, Medilax, Phenolax	Phenolphthalein	Laxative
Moduretic, Moduret	Amiloride HCl and Hydrochlorothiazide	Thiazide Diuretic, Antihypertensive
Mogadon	Nitrazepam	Benzodiazepine

Mol-Iron, Feosol, Fer-in-Sol	Ferrous Sulfate	Hematinic
Monistat I.V.	Miconazole	Antifungal
Monistat, Monistat-3, Monistat-7, Monistat Dual Pak, Feaizol, M-Zole, Micozole, Monazole	Miconazole Nitrate, Vaginal	Antifungal
Monistat-Derm, Micatin, Lotrimin-AF, Fungoid, Zeasorb-AF, Ony-Clear	Miconazole Nitrate, Topical	Antifungal
Monocid	Cefonicid	Antibiotic
Monopril	Fosinopril	Antihypertensive
Monurol	Fosfomycin Tromethamine	Urinary Anti-infective
MorphiDex	Morphine & Dextromethorphan	Cancer Pain
Motilium	Domperidone	Antiemetic
Moxam	Moxalactam	Antibiotic
MT 100	Metoclopramide and Naproxen	Oral antimigraine
Mucomyst	Acetylcysteine	Mucolytic Agent
Mucomyst 10 I.V.	Acetylcysteine Injection	Antidote
Mustargen, HN2, Nitrogen Mustard	Mechlorethamine HCl	Antineoplastic

Mutamycin, Mitoextra	Mitomycin, Mitomycin-C, MTC	Antineoplastic
Myambutol, Etibi	Ethambutol HCl	Antituberculosis Agent
Mycelex Oral Troches	Clotrimazole Lozenges	Antifungal
Mycifradin	Neomycin Sulfate	Antibiotic
Myciguent	Neomycin Ointment	Topical Antibacterial
Mycobutin	Rifabutin	Antibiotic
Mycogen-II, Mycolog-II, Mytrex, Tri-Statin II	Nystatin and Triamcinolone	Antifungal Steroid Combination
Mycostatin, Candistatin	Nystatin Vaginal	Antifungal
Mycostatin, Nilstat, , Nadostine	Nystatin Oral	Antifungal
Mycostatin, Nilstat, Nystex, Pedi-Dri, Nystop, Nyaderm	Nystatin Topical	Antifungal
Mydriacyl	Tropicamide	Cycloplegic, mydriatic
Mylanta Suspension	Aluminum Hydroxide and Magnesium Hydroxide w/ Simethicone Suspension	Antacid
Myleran	Busulfan Tab	Antineoplastic
Myloral	Bovine Myelin	Tx of MS

Mylotarg	Gemtuzumab Ozogamicin (Zogamicin)	Monoclonal antibody, Antineoplastic
Myobloc (NeuroBloc)	Botulinum Toxin, Type B	Tx of cervical dystonia (spasmodic torticollis)
Myochrysine, Aurolate	Gold Sodium Thiomalate	Antirheumatic
Myoflex, Aspercreme, Aspergel, Mobisyl, Myoflex, Exocaiae	Trolamine Salicylate	Topical Analgesic
Myoscint	Imciromab	Detecting necrosis of transplant rejection
Myotrophin	Mecasermin, Recombinant, rh-IGF-1	Neurologic Agent
Myslee	Myslee	Tx of insomnia
Mysoline, Sertan	Primidone	Anticonvulsant
Mytelase	AmbenoniumChloride	Muscle Stimulant
Nabi-HB, BayHep	Hepatitis B Immune Ghobulin (H-BIG)	Blood product
Nafcil, Nallpen, Unipen	Nafcillin Sodium	Antibiotic
Naftin	Naftifine HCl	Topical antifungal
Nalfon	Fenoprofen Calcium	Analgesic, Anti-inflammatory
Naltrel	Naltrexone Injection	Narcotic Antagonist

Naphcon, Vasocon, AK-Con, Allerest, Clear Eyes, Degest-2, VasoClear, Nafazair	Naphazoline HCl, Ophthalmic	Ophth. Vasoconstrictor
Naphcon-A, Opcon-A, Visine-A, Ocuhist	Naphazoline and Pheniramine	Ophth. Vasoconstrictor
Naprosyn, Napron X	Naproxen	Analgesic, Antiinflammatory
Naqua, Metahydrin, Aguacot, Diurese, Niazide, Trichlorex	Trichlormethiazde	Diuretic
Narcan	Naloxone HCl	Narcotic Antagonist
Nardil	Phenelzine Sulfate	Antidepressant
Naropin	Ropivacaine	Local Anesthetic
Nasacort, Azmacort	Triamcinolone Acetonide Inhaler	Anti-inflammatoy
Nasonex	Mometasone Nasal	Antiinflammatory
Natacyn	Natamycin	Ophthalmic Antifungal Agent
Natrecor	Nesiritide (B-type natriuretic peptide)	Tx of acute CHF
Naturetin	Bendroflumethiazide	Thiazide Diuretic
Navane	Thiothixene	Antipsychotic
Navelbine	Vinorelbine Tartrate	Antineoplastic

Nebcin	Tobramycin	Antibiotic
NegGram	Nalidixic Acid	Urinary Anti-infective
Nembutal, Nova Rectal	Pentobarbital Sodium	Sedative, Hypnotic
Neo-Calglucon	Calcium Glubionate	Calcium Suppliment
Neocon 1/50, Nelova 1/50M, Norinyl 1 + 50, Ortho-Novum 1/50	Mestranol and Noretrindrone	Contraceptive
Neosporin Cream	Neomycin and Polymyxjn Cream	Topical Antibacterial
Neosporin Ointment, Triple Antibiotic Oint.	Neomycin, Polymyxjn and Bacitracin Oint	Topical Antibacterial
Neosporin Ophth. Oint	Neomycin, Polymyxjn and Bacitracin Oint	Ophth. Antibacterial
Neosporin Ophth. Sol.	Neomycin, Polymyxjn and Gramicidin Ophth. Sol.	Ophth. Antibacterial
Neosten	Sodium Fluoride Extended Release	Tx of osteoporosis
NeoStrata AHA Gel, Solaquin Forte, Nuquin HP	Hydroquinone Gel	Skin Bleach
Neo-Synephrine	Phenylephrine HCl Injection	Vasopressor
Neo-Synephrine	Phenylephrine HCl Nasal Solution	Adrenergic, Decongestant, Sympathomimetic, Vasoconstrictor

Neo-Synephrine, Mydfrin, Relies	Phenylephrine HCl Ophthalmic Solution	Adrenergic, Mydriatic, Sympathomimetic, Vasoconstrictor
NeoTect	TechnetiumTc99m depreotide	Imaging agent
Neotrofin	Leteprinim Potassium	Tx of Alzheimer's Disease
Neptazane, GlaucTabs	Methazolamide	Antiglaucoma
Nesacaine	Chloroprocaine	Local Anesthetic
Netromycin	Netilmicin	Antibiotic
Neumega (rh-IL-11)	Oprelvekin (Recombinant Interleukin-11)	Tx of Chemotherapy induced thrombocytopenia
Neupogen Sustained Release	Pegfilgrastim	Stimulate WBC formation
Neupogen, G-CSF	Figrastim	Stimulate WBC formation
Neuprex	Opebecan	Antibacterial
Neurelan	Fampridine	Tx of multiple sclerosis
NeuroCell-PD	Porcine fetal cell transplant	Tx of Parkinson's Disease
Neurontin	Gabapentin	Anticonvulsant
Neutralase	Heparinase I	Antithrombotic
Neutrexin	Trimetrexate Glucuronate	Antiparasitic, antineoplastic
Nexium	Esomeprazole Magnesium	Supress Gastric Acid Secretion
Niacin, Nicotinic Acid	Vitamin B3	Vitamin

NicErase-SL	Lobeline	Smoking Deterrent
Niclocide	Niclosamide	Anthelminic
Nicobid, Nicolar, Nicotinex	Nicotinic Acid (Niacin)	Vitamin, Peripheral Vasodilator, Antihyperlipidemic
Nicobid, Nicolar, Nicotinex, Nispan, SloNiacin	Niacin (Nicotinic Acid)	Vitamin, Peripheral Vasodilator, Antihyperlipidemic
Nicorette, Nicotrol-DS	Nicotine Polacrilex	Smoking Deterrent
Niferex	Ferrous Polysaccharide	Hematinic
Nilandron, Anadron	Nilutamide	Antiandrogen
Nimbex	Cisatracurium Besylate	Skeletal Muscle Relaxant
Nimotop	Nimodipine	Calcium Channel Blocker, for Subarachnoid Hemorrhage (SAH)
Nipent	Pentostatin (2'-deoxycoformycin, DCF)	Antineoplastic
Nipride, Nitropress	Nitroprusside Sodium	I.V. Antihypertensive
Nitro-Bid, Nitrostat, Tridil, Nitrolingual, Nitrogard, Nitrong, Nitroglyn, Nitrocine, Nitro-Time	Nitroglycerin	Antianginal Agent

Nitrol, Nitro-Bid	Nitroglycerin Ointment	Antianginal Agent
Nizoral, Nizoral AD	Ketoconazole	Antifungal
Noctec, Aquachloral, Somnote	Chloral Hydrate	Sedative Hypnotic, Anxiolytic
NoDoz, Vivarin, Caffedrine, Stay Awake, Quick-Pep	Caffeine	CNS Stimulant
Nolahist	Phenindamine Tartrate	Antihistamine
Nolvadex, Tamofen, Tamone	Tamoxifen Citrate	Adjunct to breast surgery in Tx of breast cancer
Norco	Hydrocodone with Acetaminophen	Narcotic analgesic
Norcuron	Vecuronium Bromide	Skeletal muscle relaxant
Norflex, Banflex, Felxoject, Myolin, Flexon	Orphenadrine Citrate	Skeletal Muscle Relaxant
Norgesic, Norgesic-Forte	Orphenadrine Citrate, ASA and Caffeine	Analgesic, Muscle Relaxant combination
Noritate, MetroGel,	Metronidazole Topical	Antiinfective
Normiflo	Ardeparin	Low molecular weight heparin
Normix	Rifaximin	Hepatic encephalopathy

Normodyne, Trandate	Labetalol HCl	Antihypertensive
Normosang	Heme Arginate	Tx of acute porphyria
Noroxin	Norfloxacin Oral	Antibiotic
Norpace, Norpace-CR, Rythmodan-LA	Disopyramide Phosphate	Antiarrhythmic
Norplant	Levonorgestrel	Implant Contraceptive
Norpramin, Pertofrane	Desipramine HCl	Antidepressant
Norvasc	Amlodipine Besylate	Calcium Channel Blocker, Antihypertensive
Norvir	Ritonavir	Antiviral
Novantrone	Mitoxantrone HCl	Antineoplastic
Novastan, ACOVA	Argatroban	Selective Thrombin Inhibitor-Anticoagulant
Novocaine	Procaine HCl	Local Anesthetic
NovoRapid	Insulin Aspart	Hormone
NovoSeven, NiasStase	Factor VII, Recombinant	Treatment of hemophilia A or B
Nubain	Nalbuphine HCl	Narcotic Agonist-Antagonist Analgesic
Numorphan	Oxymorphone HCl	Narcotic Analgesic
Nupercainal	Dibucaine	Topical Anesthetic
Nuromax	Doxacurium Cl	Nondepolarizing Neuromuscular Blocker

Nutropin Depot	Somatropin Depot	Long acting dosage form of Recombinant Growth Hormone (rhGH)
Nutropin, Genotropin, Humatrope, Saizen, Norditropin, ProLease, Serostim (rh-GH), Nutropin Depot, Siazen	Somatropin	Growth Hormone
Nydrazid, Laniazid	Isoniazid (INH)	Antituberculosis
Nydrazid, Laniazid, Isotamine	INH (Isoniazid)	Antituberculosis
Nyotran	Nystatin Injection	Antifungal
OcuClear, Visine LR	Oxymetazoline HCl Ophthalmic	Ophthalmic Vasoconstrictor
Ocufen	Flurbiprofen Sodium	Antiinflammatory
Ocuflox	Ofloxacin Opthalmic	Ophthalmic Antibiotic
Ocupress	Carteolol Ophthalmic	Antiglaucoma
Ogen, Ortho-Est, Estropipate	Estropipate (Piperazine Estrone Sulfate)	Hormone, Estrogen
Olux	Clobetasol Topical Foam	Topical Anti-inflammitory, Corticosteroid
Omnicef	Cefdinir	Antibiotic

Omniferon	Multisubtype alpha interferon	Tx of hepatitis C
Omnipaque	Iohexol	Diagnostic Aid
Omnipen, Principen, Totacillin, Polycillin, Ampicin, Penbritin	Ampicillin	Antibiotic
OncoLAR	Octreotide Pamoate	Hormone Inhibitor
Onconase	Ranpirnase	Antineoplastic
Oncovin, Vincasar, VCR	Vincristine Sulfate	Antineoplastic
Onkolox	Coumarin	Tx of renal cell carcinoma
Ontak	Denileukin difitox	Cutaneous t-cell lymphoma (CTCL)
Opthaine, Opthetic, Alcaine	Proparacaine	Local Anesthetic
Opticrom, Crolom	Cromolyn Ophth Sol	EENT Misc. Drug
Optimark	Gadoversetamide	MRI Contrast Agent
Optimine	Azatadine Maleate	Antihistamine
Optipranolol	Metipranolol HCl	Antiglaucoma Agent
Optiray 160	Ioversol 34%	Diagnostic Aid
Optiray 240	Ioversol 51%	Diagnostic Aid
Optiray 320	Ioversol 68%	Diagnostic Aid
Optivar	Azelastine Opthalmic	Antihistamine
Oragrafin Calcium	Ipodate Calcium	Diagnostic Aid

Orajel Perioseptic, Proxigel	Carbamide Peroxide (Urea Peroxide)	Tx of oral inflammation
Orap	Pimozide	Antipsychotic
Oreton Methyl, Android, Testred, Virilon, Methitest, Metandren	Methyltestosterone	Anabolic Steroid
Orgaran	Danaparoid Sodium	Anticoagulant,LMWH
Orgotein	Superoxide Dismutase (bovine)	Tx of ALS
Orimune	Poliovirus Vaccine	Vaccine
Orinase, Tol-Tab	Tolbutamide	Antidiabetic
Orlaam	Levomethadyl acetate	Tx of opiate addiction
Ornidyl	Eflornithine HCl	Antiprotozoal, Tx of trypanosoma brucei gambiense infection (sleeping sickness)
Ortho Dienestrol, DV	Dienestrol	Estrogen
Orthoclone OKT3	Muromonab-CD3	Immunosuppressant
Ortho-Prefest, 17ß-Estradiol & Norgestimate	Estradiol/Norgestimate	Hormone Replacement
Orudis, Oruvail, Actron, Orafen, Orudis KT (OTC)	Ketoprofen	Analgesic, Antiinflammitory
Orzel	Tegafur & Leucovorin	Antineoplastic for metastatic colorectal cancer

319

Osmitrol, Resectisol	Mannitol	Osmotic Diuretic
Osmoglyn	Glycerin (Glycerol)	Osmotic Diuretic
Ostac	Clodronate Disodium	Bisphosphonate
Osteo-D	Secalciferol	Familial hypophosphatemic rickets
Otrivin, Inspire, Chlorohist-LA, Neo-Synephrine II Long Acting	Xylometazoline	Nasal Decongestant
Ovastat	Treosulfan	Tx of ovarian cancer
Ovide Lotion	Malathion Lotion	Pediculicide, Tx of lice, Scabicide
Ovidrel	Choriogonadotropin alfa for Injection	Ovulation Induction
Ovrette	Norgestrel	Contraceptive
Oxandrin, Hepandrin	Oxandrolone	Anabolic Steroid
Oxistat, Oxizole	Oxiconazole	Antifungal
Oxsodrol	Superoxide Dismutase (recombinant human)	Prevention of reperfusion injury to donor organ tissue
Oxsoralen	Methoxsalen Topical	Repigmenting agent in vitiligo
Oxsoralen-Ultra, 8-MOP	Methoxsalen Oral	Treatment of psoriasis, Repigmentation of idiopathic vitiligo.
Oxygent	Perflubron	Oxygen Carrier

	Emulsion	
OxyIR, OxyContin, Roxicodone, OxyFast, M-Oxy, Percolone, Roxicodone SR, Endocodone, Supeudol	Oxycodone HCl	Narcotic aqnalgesic
P_E_, E-Pilo	Pilocarpine & Epinephrine	Antiglaucoma
Pacis	BCG, Live	Immunotherapy
Pagaclone	Pagaclone	Tx of panic disorder
Pamine	Methscopolamine Bromide	GI Anticholinergic, Antispasmotic
Pandel	Hydrocortisone Buteprate	Topical Antiinflammatory
Panhematin	Hemin	Tx of porphyria
Panlor-DC	Acetaminophen, Caffeine and Dihydrocodeine	Analgesic combination
Panorex	Edrecolomab	Tx of colon and rectal cancer
Panretin Gel	Alitretinoin (LGD1057)	Cutaneous lesions with AIDS related Kaposi's sarcoma
Panthoderm Cream	Dexpanthenol Topical	Relief of pruritis
Pantothenic Acid	Vitamin B5	Vitamin
Paradione	Paramethadione	Anticonvulsant

Parafon Forte DSC, Paraflex, Remular-S	Chlorzoxazone	Skeletal Muscle Relaxant
Paral	Paraldehyde	Sedative Hypnotic
Paraplatin	Carboplatin	Antineoplastic
Paregoric	Camphorated Tincture of Opium	Antiperistaltic, Narcotic
Paregoric	Opium Tincture, Camphorated	Narcotic
Parlodel	Bromocriptine Mesylate	Antiparkinson Agent
Parnate	Tranylcypromine	Antidepressant
Parsidol	Ethopropazine HCl	
Paser Granules, PAS	Aminosalicylic Acid	Tx of Tuberculosis infections
Paser, Sodium P.A.S., Teebacin, Tubasal	Aminosalicylate Sodium	Tx of Tuberculosis infections
Pasmanate, Plasma-Plex, Protenate, Plasmatein	Plasma Protein Fraction	Hypoproteinemia, Plasma Volume Expander
Patanol	Olopatadine	Ophth. Antihistamine
Pavabid. Genabid, Pavatine	Papaverine HCl	Peripheral Vasodilator
Pavulon	Pancuronium Bromide	Muscle Relaxant
Paxarel	Acetylcarbromal	Hypnotic, Sedative
Paxi, Paxil CRl	Paroxetine HCl	Antidepressant, Tx of OCD/panic disorder/ social phobia

Paxipam	Halazepam	Anxiolytic
PBZ, Tripelennamine, Tebrazid	Pyribenzamine	Antihistamine (H1)
Pediastat	Miconazole Nitrate low concentration, Topical	Tx of diaper dermatitis
Pediazole	Erythromycin Ethylsuccinate and Sulfisoxazole	Antibiotic
Peganone	Ethotoin	Anticonvulsant
Peg-Intron (Pegasys) (PEG-IFN alfa-2a, Pegylated Interfon alfa-2a)	Peginterferon alfa-2a	Tx of Hepatitis C, also Tx of CML & Renal Ca
Penetrex	Enoxacin	Antibiotic
Penicillin-G Sodium	Penicillin-G Sodium (Aqueous) Parenteral	Antibiotic
Penlac	Ciclopirox Nail Lacquer	Antifungal
Pentam, Nebupent, Pentacarinat	Pentamidine Isethionate	Misc. Anti-infective
Pentasa, Asacol	Mesalamine Oral	Bowel Anti-inflammatory
Pentaspan	Pentastarch	Harvesting Aid
Pentavac	Pentavalent Vaccine	Vaccine
Penthrane	Methoxyflurane	Inhalant Anesthetic
Pentids	Penicillin-G Potassium Oral	Antibiotic

Pentosam	Sodium antimony gluconate (Sodium stibogluconate)	Antiinfective
Pentothal	Thiopental	Anesthetic
Pepatavon	Pentagastrin	Diagnostic Aid
Pepcid Complete	Famotidine, Calcium Carbonate, Magnesium Hydroxide	Combination antacid and H-2 blocker
Pepcid, Pepcid-AD, Mylanta-AR, Pepcid-RDP	Famotidine	Anti-ulcer
Pepto-Bismol	Bismuth Subsalicylate	Misc. GI Agent
Perchloracap (not intended for intravascular Admin)	Potassium Perchlorate	Diagnostic Aid
Percocet, Roxicet, Tylox, Roxilox, Endocet	Oxycodone HCl, Acetaminophen	Narcotic Analgesic
Percodan, Roxiprin	Oxycodone HCl & Aspirin	Narcotic Analgesic
Percogesic, Phenylgesic	Phenyltoloxamine Citrate & Acetaminophen	Antihistamine Analgesic Combination
Perfan	Enoximone	Tx of heart failure
Periactin	Cyproheptadine	Antihistamine
Pericolace, DSS+, Doxidan	Docusate Sodium with Casanthranol	Laxative, stool softener
Peridex, Periogard, Oro Clense	Chlorhexidine Gluconate Oral	Topical Antiinfective

Peritrate, Pentylan, PETN	Pentaerythritol Tetranitrate	Nitrate
Permax	Pergolide Mesylate	Antiparkinson Abent
Persantine	Dipyridamole	Platelet Aggregation Inhibitor
Pfizerpen	Penicillin-G Potassium (Aqueous), Parenteral	Antibiotic
Phenerbel-S, Belergal-S, Folergot DF	L-Alkaloids of Belladonna, Phenobarbital and Ergotamine Tartrate	GI-Antichohinergic, Antispasmotic
Phenergan	Promethazine	Antihistamine, Antiemetic
Phenurone	Phenacemide	Anticonvulsant
Phenylase	Phenylalanine ammonia-lyase	Hyperphenylalaninemia
PhosLo, Cahphron	Calcium Acetate	Tx of Hyperphosphatemia in Endstage Renal Disease
Phospholine Iodide	Echothiophate Iodide	Antiglaucoma, Miotic
Photofrin	Porfimer sodium	Tx of certain carcinomas
Phrenilin	Butalbital and Acetaminophen	Analgesic
Phrilamine Maleate	Pyrilamine Maleate	Antihistamine
Phytonadione	Vitamin K1	Vitamin, Hemostatic

Pilagan	Pilocarpine Nitrate	Antiglaucoma
Pindac	Pinacidil	Antihypertensive
Pin-Rid, Antiminth, Combantrin, Pin-X, Reese's Pinworm	Pyrantel Pamoate	Anthelminic
Pipracil	Piperacillin Sodium	Antibiotic
Pitocin, Syntocinon	Oxytocin	Oxytocic
Pitressin, ADH	Vasopressin (8-Arginine Vasopressin)	For Diabetes Insipidus, Tx of variceal bleeding
Placidyl	Ethchlorvynol	Hypnotic, Sedative
Plague Vaccine	Plague Vaccine	Vaccine
Plan B, Levonelle (UK)	Levonorgestrel (Progestin)	Prevention of pregnancy after unprotected sex.
Plaquenil	Hydroxychloroquine Sulfate	Antimalarial, Antirheumatic
Platinol	Cisplatin	Antineoplastic
Plavix	Clopidogrel	Platelet Aggregation Inhibitor
Plegine, Bontril-PDM, Adipost, Dital, Melfiat, Prelu-2, Rexigen, Dyrexan-OD, Melfiat	Phendimetrazine Tartrate	Anorexiant
Plendil, Renedil	Felodipine	Calcium Channel Blocker, Antihypertensive

Pletal	Cilostazol	Platelet Inhibitor
PMPA, Tenofovir	Tenofovir Disoproxil Fumarate	Antiretroviral Agent
Pneumovax, Pnu-Imune, Pneumo-23	Pneumococcal Vaccine	Vaccine
Podocon-25, Podofin, Podofilm	Podophyllin	Antiviral
Polaramine	Dexchlorpheniramine Maleate	Antihistamine
Polycillin-PRB, Probampacin	Ampicillin with Probenecid	Antibiotic
Polycitra, Polycitra-LC	Potassium Citrate, Sodium Citrate & Citric Acid	Urinary Alkalinizer
Polycitra-K	Potassium Citrate & Citric Acid	Urinary Alkalinizer
Polysporin Ophth.Oint.	Polymyxin B & Bacitracin Ophth. Oint.	Ophth. Antibacterial
Polysporin, Double Antibiotic Ointment, Polysporin Powder, Polysporin Spray	Bacitracin and Polymyxin	Topical Antibacterial
Polytrim Ophth. Sol.	Trimethoprim & Polymyxin-B Ophth	EENT Anti-infective
Pondimin	Fenfluramine	Anorexiant
Ponstel	Mefanamic Acid	Analgesic

Pontocaine	Tetracaine	Local Anesthetic
Pontocaine Ophth.	Tetracaine Ophth.	Topical Anesthetic
Posture	Tribasic Calcium Phosphate	Calcium Suppliment
PPD, Aplisol, Tubersol, Mantoux	Tuberculin Injection	TB Skin Test
Prandin, Gluconorm	Repaglinide	Antidiabetic (meglitinide class)
Pravachol	Pravastatin	Antihyperlipidemic
Precedex	Dexmedetomidine	Sedation Induction
Precef	Ceforanide	Antibiotic, cephalosporin
Precose, Prandase	Acarbose	Antidiabetic
Pred Mild, Pred Forte, Econopred, AK-Pred, Inflamase	Prednisolone Ophth.	Corticosteroid
Prelone, Delta-Cortef	Prednisolone	Glucocorticoid
Premarin	Conjugated Estrogens	Hormone Replacement
Premarin	Estrogens, Conjugated	Hormone
Premarin with Methyltestosterone	Estrogens with Methyltestosterone	Hormone
Premesis-Rx	B6, Folic Acid, B12, and Calcium Carbonate	Tx of pregnancy induced nausea
Premphase	Conjugated Estrogens, Medroxyprogestero	Estrogen Progestin Combination

	ne Acetate Combination	
Prempro	Medroxyprogesterone Acetate & Conjugated Estrogens	Estrogen Progestin Combination
Prempro, Prempro Low Dose	Conjugated Estrogens, Medroxyprogesterone Acetate	Estrogen Progestin Combination
Pretz-D, Kondon's Nasal	Ephedrine Nasal	Nasal Decongestant
Prevacid	Lansoprazole	Supress Gastric Acid Secretion
Preven	Ethinyl Estradiol and Levonorgestrel	Prevention of pregnancy after unprotected sex.
Preveon	Adefovir Dipivoxil	Antiviral, NRTI
Prevnar	Pneumococcal 7-Valent Conjugate Vaccine	Vaccine
Priftin	Rifapentine	Antibiotic, Tx of Tuberculosis
Prilosec	Omeprazole	Supress Gastric Acid Secretion
Primacor	Milrinone Lactate	Inotropic/vasodialtor
Primaquine	Primaquine Phosphate	Antimalarial
Primaxin	Imipenem-Cilastatin	Antibiotic

Prinivil, Zestril	Lisinopril	Antihypertensive
Prinzide, Zestoretic	Lisinopril and Hydrochlorothiazide	Antihypertensive
Priscoline	Tolazoline	Antihypertensive
Privine	Naphazoline HCl, Nasal	Nasal Decongestant
ProAmatine	Midodrine	Alpha-1 agonist, for orthostatic hypotention
Pro-Banthine	Propantheline Bromine	Anticholinergic, Antispasnodic
Procardia, Adalat, Procardia-XL, Adalat-CC, Nifedical XL	Nifedipine	Calcium Channel Blocker, Antianginal, Antihypertensive (SR Only)
Proderm Topical	Castor Oil and Balsam of Peru	Prevent and Tx of decubitus Ulcers
Profenal	Suprofen	Antiinflammatory
Progestasert	Progesterone Intrauterine	Contraceptive
Proglycem	Diazoxide Oral	Hyperglycemic
Prograf, FK506	Tacrolimus	Immunosupressant
Prolastin	Alpha-1-Proteinase Inhibitor (Human)	Tx of alpha-1 antitrypsin deficiency
Prolastin	Alpha-1-Proteinase Inhibitor (Human)	Emphysema
Proleukin, Interleukin-2	Aldesleukin IL-2	Biologic Response Modifier
Prolixin Decanoate	Fluphenazine Decanoate	Antipsychotic

Prolixin Enanthate	Fluphenazine Enanthate	Antipsychotic
Prolixin, Permitil	Fluphenazine HCl	Antipsychotic
Proloprim, Trimpex, Primsol	Trimethoprim	Urinary Anti-infective
ProLyse	Prourokinase, Recombinant	Thrombolytic
Promega, Max EPA, Fish Oil	Omega-3-fatty acids	Dietary suppliment
ProMem, Trichlorfon	Metrifonate	Treatment of Alzheimer's Disease
Prometrium, Crinone Vag. Gel	Progesterone, Micronized	Progestin
Promycin	Porfiromycin	Antineoplastic
Pronemia Hematinic Capsules	Hematinic Concentrate with Intrinsic Factor	Hematinic
Pronestyl, Procan, Pronestyl-SR, Procan-SR	Procainamide HCl	Group I-A Antiarrhythmic
Propadrine, Rhindecon, Propagest, Acutrim, Dexatrim, Phenyldrine	Phenylpropanolamine HCl	Nasal Decongestant, Anorexiant
Propine	Dipivefrin HCl	Antiglaucoma, Midriatic
Propulsid	Cisapride	Antiemetic, Prokinetic Agent, GI Stimulant

Propylthiouracil (PTU)	Propylthiouracil	Tx of hyperthyroidism and/or large goiters.
Proscar, Propecia	Finasteride	BPH Drug (Proscar) Hair Growth Stimulator (Propecia)
Prosed/DS	Methenamine, Phenyl Salicylate, Atropine, Hyoscyamine, Benzoic acid and Methylene Blue,	Urinary analgesic
Prosom	Estazolam	Sedative/hypnotic
Prostaphlin, Bactocill	Oxacillin Sodium	Antibiotic
Prostigmin	Neostigmine	Cholinergic Muscle Stimulant
Prostin VR Pediatric	Alprostadil (PGE1 Prostaglandin E1)	Tx of ductus arteriosus until surgery
Prostin-E2, Prepidel, Cervidil, PGE2	Dinoprostone	Agents for cervical ripening
Protamine Sulfate	Protamine Sulfate	Heparin Antagonist
Protara	Acadesine	For MI prophylaxis
ProTec, LSF	Lisofylline	Immunomodulator
ProTech First Aid Stik	Povidone-Iodide And Lidocaine	Cleaning and pain relief of cuts, scrapes and burns
Prothiaden	Dothiepin HCl	Tricyclic Antidepressant
Protonix	Pantoprazole	Supress Gastric Acid Secretion

Protopam Chloride	Pralidoxime Chloride (2-PAM)	Antidote
Protopic	Tacrolimus Ointment	Tx of atopic dermatitis (eczema)
Protropin	Somatrem	Growth Hormone
Provatene	Beta-Carotene	Vitamin A precursor
Proventil, Ventolin, Volmax, Proventil HFA, AccuNeb	Albuterol Sulfate	Bronchodilator
Provera, Cycrin, Amen, Curretab	Medroxyprogesterone Acetate	Hormone, Progestin
Provigil, Alertec	Modafinil	For Narcolepsy
Prozac Weekly Capsules	Fluoxetine Extended Release	Antidepressant, SSRI
Prozac, Sarafem	Fluoxetine	Antidepressant, Tx of OCD, Tx of bulimia (60mg/day) SSRI
Pulmicort Respules	Budesonide Suspension	Asthma
Pulmicort Turbuhaler	Budesonide Inhalation Powder	Antiinflammatory, Antiasthmatic
Pulmozyme	Dornase Alfa	Respirtory Enzyme
Purinethol, 6-MP	Mercaptopurine	Antineoplastic
Purlytin	Tin ethyl etiepurpurin	Tx of macular degeneration
Pyribenzamine, PBZ, Pelamine, Triplen, Vaginex	Tripelennamine	Antihistamine

Pyridium Plus	Phenazopyridine, Hyoscyamine HBr, Butalbital	Urinary Analgesic
Pyridium, UTI Relief Urodine, Azo-Standard, Prodium, Baridium, Geridiium, Pyridiate, Urogesic, Urodol, Viridium, Pyronium, Phenazo tab	Phenazopyridine HCl	Urinary Analgesic
Pyridoxine	Vitamin B6	Vitamin
Quadramet	Samarium 153	Antineoplastic
Quarzan	Clidinium Bromide	GI Anticholinergic, Antispasmodic
Quelicin, Anectine, Sucostrin	Succinylcholine Chloride	Neuromuscular Blocking Agent
Questran	Qholestyramine Resin	Antilipemic
Questran, Questran Light, Prevalite, LoCHOLEST Light, LoCHOLEST	Cholestyramine	Antilipemic
Quilimmune-P	Pneumococcal Polysaccharide Vaccine	Vaccine

Quinamm, M-KYA, Formula Q	Quinine Sulfate	Antimalarial
Quinate,Quinaglute Dura-Tabs, Quinalan	Quinidine Gluconate	Group I-A Antiarrhythmic
Quinora, Quinidex Extentabs	Quinidine Sulfate	Group I-A Antiarrhythmic
Quixin	Levofloxacin Ophthalmic Solution	Opthalmic Antibiotic
RabAvert	Rabies Vaccine	Vaccine
Radinyl	Ethanidazole	Chemosensitizer, Radiosensitizer
Ramoplanin Oral	Ramoplanin	Antibacterial
Ramses, Koromex, Because, Conceptrol, Emko, Delfen, Gynol II, Encare, Ortho-Gynol, Semicid, Advantge-S	Nonoxynol 9 Vaginal Jelly	Spermicide Contraceptive
Rapamune (Rapamycin)	Sirolimus	Anti-rejection
Raplon	Rapacuronium Bromide	Nondepolarizing neuromuscular blocking agent
Raudixin, Rauval	Rauwolfia Serpentia	Antihypertensive, Antipsychotic
Rauzide	Rauwolfia Serpentia & Bendroflumethiazid	Antihypertensive

	e	
Ravocaine & Novocaine with Levophed	Propoxycaine & Procaine with Norepinephrine	Local Anesthetic
Raxar	Grepafloxacin	Antibiotic
Rebetron, Rebetol	Ribavirin Caps & Interferon alfa-2b Inj.	Antiviral
Rebif	Interferon Beta-1a, Recombinant, rh-INF-beta	Neurologic Agent
Redux	Desfenfluramine	Anorexiant
ReFacto, Bioclate, Helixate,Recombinate, Alphanate, Hemofil, Humate,Hyate,Koate, Monoclate, Profilate, Kogenate, Monarc-M	Antihemophilic Factor, AHF, Factor VIII	Tx of hemophilia-A
Refludan	Lepirudin-DNA	Hirudin, Thrombin Inhibitor-Anticoagulant
Regitine, Vasomax, Rogitine	Phentolamine Mesylate	Antihypertensive, Sympatholytic
Reglan, Clopra, Maxolon, Octamide, Reclomide	Metoclopramide HCl	Prokinetic agent, antinausea
Regranex	Becaplermin	Misc. Skin Product

	Topical	
Regroton	Chlorthalidone & Reserpine	Antihypertensive
Relafen	Nabumetone	Analgesic, Anti-inflammitory
Relenza	Zanamivir	Antiviral (Neuraminidase Inhibitor)
Relpax	Eletriptan	Antimigraine
Remeron, Remeron SolTab	Mirtazapine	Antidepressant (Tetracyclic)
Remicade, cA2	Infliximab	Treatment of Chron's Disease, Rheumatoid Arthritis, Psoriasis
RemiFemin	Black Cohosh Extact	Tx of menopause
Reminyl, Nivalin	Galantamine HBr	Acetylcholinesterase Inhibitor for Tx of Alzheimer's
Remodulin, Uniprost	UT-15	Tx of pulmonary arterial hypertension
Removue-Dip	Iodamide Meglumine 24%	Diagnostic Aid
Remune	Immune-based Whole Inactivated HIV-1 Virus	HIV Antiviral Vaccine
Renagel	Sevelamer HCl	Hyperphosphatemia of end stage renal disease
Renese	Polythiazide	Diuretic
Renese-R	Reserpine and	Antihypertensive

	Polythiazide	
Renova, Avita, Retin-A, Vesanoid, Altinac (ATRA), Retisel-A, Stievaa	Tretinoin	Dermatologic
Renovist	Diatrizoate Meglumine 34.3% and Diatrizoate Sodium 35%	Diagnostic Aid
Renovist II	Diatrizoate Meglumine 28.5% and diatrizoate Sodium 29.1%	Diagnostic Aid
Renovue-65	Iodamide Meglumine 65%	Diagnostic Aid
ReoPro	Abciximab	Antiplatelet
Repronex, Pergonal, Humegon	Menotropins for Injection (Gonadotropins,	A human gonadotropin product
Requip	Ropinirole HCl	Antiparkinsonian
Rescriptor	Delavirdine Mesylate	Antiviral
Rescula	Unoprostone Isopropyl Ophthalmic Solution	Tx of open-angle glaucoma or ocular hypertention
Resectisol	Mannitol Irrigation	Hexitol Irrigants
RespiGam, Respivir	RSV Immune Globulin	Immunoglobulin
Restasis	Cyclosporine Ophth. Emulsion	Dry eye disease
Restoril	Temazepam	Sedative, Hypnotic

Retavase	Reteplase (rPA)	Thrombolytic
Retrovir, AZT, ZDV	Zidovudine (Azidothymidine, Compound S)	Antiviral
Revasc	Desirudin (Recombinant Hirudin)	Prevention of deep vein thrombosis after hip replacement surgery
Revasc	Hirudin	Direct Thrombin Inhibitor-Anticoagulant
Revex, Cervene	Nalmefene HCl	Narcotic Antagonist
ReVia, Depade, Trexan	Naltrexone HCl	Narcotic Antagonist
Rezulin	Troglitazone	Antidiabetic, (thiazolidinedione)
rhATIII	Recombinant Human Antithrombin III	To restore heparin sensitivity in resistant patients prior to bypass surgery
Rheomacrodex, Gentran, Macrodex	Dextran	Plasma Volume Expander
Rhinocort Aqua	Budesonide, Aqua	Nasal Anti-inflammatory
Rhinocort, Rhinocort Aqua	Budesonide	Nasal Anti-inflammatory
RhoGAM, BayRho-D, WinRho SDF, Gamulin Rh, HypRho-D	RHO Immune Globulin	Immunoglobulin

Riboflavin	Vitamin B2	Vitamin
Ridaura	Auranofin	Antirheumatic
Rifamate	Rifampin and Isoniazid	Antitubercular
Rifater	Rifampin, Isoniazid and Pyrazinamide	Tx of tuberculosis
Rilutek	Riluzole	Treatment of Amylotrophic Lateral Sclerosis (ALS)(Lou Gehrig's Disease)
Rimactane, Rifidin, Rofact, Rimycin	Rifampin	Antibiotic
Rimadyl	Carprofen	Anti-inflammatory, analgesic
Rimso-50, DMSO	Dimethyl Sulfoxide	Interstitial Cystitis
Riopan	Magaldrate	Antacid
Risperdal	Risperidone	Antipsychotic
Risperdal-LA	Risperidone	Antipsychotic
Ritalin, Metadate ER, Methylin, Concerta, Methylin ER, Riphenidaze	Methylphenidate HCl	CNS Stimulant
Rituxan	Rituximab	Antineoplastic
Rizaben	Tranilast	Prevention of restenosis after angioplasty
Robaxin	Methocarbamol	Skeletal Muscle Relaxant

Robaxisal	Methocarbamol & Aspirin	Skeletal Muscle Relaxant and Analgesic
Robinul	Glycopyrrolate	Antimuscarinic, Antispasmotic
Robitussin-AC, Tussi Organidin NR, Tussi Organibin-S NR, Guiatuss-AC	Guaifenesin and Codeine	Expectorant Antitussive
Robitussin-DM, Fenesin-DM, Humabid-DM, Tussi Organidin DM NR, Tussi Organidin DM-S NR	Guaifenesin and Dextromethorphan	Expectorant antitussive
Rocephin	Ceftriaxone	Antibiotic
Roferon-A	Interferon Alfa-2a	Antineoplastic
Rogaine	Minoxidil Topical	Stimulate Hair Growth
Romazicon, Anexate	Flumazenil	Reversal of Benzodiazepines
Rondec Oral Drops, Carbinoxamine Drops	Carbinoxamine & Pseudoephedrine	Antihistamine & Decongestant
RotaShield	Tetravalent rhesus-based rotavirus vaccine (RRV-TV)	Prevention of gastroenteritis
Rowasa	Mesalamine Rectal	Bowel Anti-inflammatory

Roxiam	Remoxipride	Antipsychotic Agent
Roxin	Roxatidine Acetate	Tx of peptic ulcers
Rubex, Adriamycin, Doxil	Doxorubicin HCl	Antineoplastic
Rythmol	Propafenone HCl	Group I-C Antiarrhythmic
Sabril	Vigabatrin	Anticonvulsant
Salagen	Pilocarpine HCl Oral	Cholinergic Parasympathomimetic
Salbutamol Ultrahaler	Salbutamol	Tx of bronchial asthma
Saleto Tablets	APAP, Aspirin, Salicylamide and caffeine	Analgesil
Salprofen	Ibuprofen Injection	Prevention/Tx of patent ductus arteriosus
Salutensin, Salutensin-Demi	Hydroflumethiazide and Reserpine	Antihypertensive
Sandimmune, Neoral, Gengraf, SangCYA	Cyclosporine (Cyclosporine-A)	Immunosuppressant
Sandostatin, Sandostatin LAR Depot	Octreotide Acetate	Tx of variceal bleeding Tx of AIDS diarrhea
Sanorex, Mazanor	Mazindol	Anorexiant, Sympathomimetic
Sansert	Methysergide Maleate	Antimigraine
Santyl	Collagenase Topical	Topical Debriding Agent

Scarlet Red Ointment Dressings	Scarlet Red Dressings	Epithelialization of donor sites, burns and wounds
Scleromate, Sodium Morrhuate	Morrhuate Sodium	Sclerosing Agent
Seconal	Secobarbital Sodium	Sedative, Hypnotic
Sectral, Monitan	Acebutolol	Antihypertensive, ß-Adrenergic Blocker, Group II Antiarrhythmic
Seldane	Terfenadine	Non-Sedating Antihistamine
Seldane-D	Terfenadine & Pseudoephrine HCl	Antihistamine, decongestant combination
Selecor	Celiprolol HCl	Tx of hypertension and angina
Selsun, Sellsun Blue, Exsel, Versel	Selenium Sulfide	Antiseborrheic, Antifungal
Senokot, Senolax, Senokotxtra	Senna	Laxative
Septocaine	Articaine HCl with Epinephrine	Local Anesthesia
Septopal	Gentamicin impregnated surgical wire	Antiinfective
Ser-Ap-Es, Cam-Ap-Es, Tri-Hydroserpine, Serpazide, Ser-A-Gen	Hydralazine, HCTZ, and Reserpine	Antihypertensive

Serax, Zapex, Novoxapam, Oxpam	Oxazepam	Sedative, Anxiolytic
Serentil	Mesoridazine	Antipsychotic
Serevent Diskus	Salmeterol Xinafoate Powder for Inhalation	Bronchodilator
Serevent Inhaler	Salmeterol Xinafoate Inhaler	Bronchodilator
Serlect	Sertindole	Antipsychotic Agent
Seromycin	Cycloserine	Antituberculosis Drug
Seroquel	Quetiapine Fumarate	Antipsychotic
Serpasil	Reserpine	Antihypertensive
Serzone	Nefazodone HCl	Antidepressant
Shur-Clens	Poloxamer 188	Protective Dressing
Sibelium	Flunarizine	Tx of alternating hemiplegia
Silvadene, SSD, Dermazin	Silver Sulfadiazine	Topical Antibacterial
Simdax	Levosimendan	Calcium sensitizer
Simulect	Basiliximab	Immunosuppressive
Sinemet, Sinemes-SR, Atamet	Carbidopa & Levodoopa	Antiparkinson agent
Sinequan, Zonalon, Triadapin	Doxepin HCl	Antidepressant
Singulair	Montelukast Sodium	Antiasthmatic

Sinografin (not intended for intravascular admin)	Diatrizoate Meglumine 52.7% and Iodipamide Meglumine 26.8%	Diagnostic Aid
Sitzmarks	Radiopaque Polyvinyl Chloride	Diagnostic Aid
Skelaxin	Metaxalone	Skeletal Muscle Relaxant
Skelid	Tiludronate	Bone Stabilizer
Slow-Mag	Magnesium Chloride	Replacement Preparation
Smart M195	Humanized M195 antibody	Tx of acute myeloid leukemia
SMART M197	Anti-CD33 monoclonal antibody	Tx of acute myeloid leukemia
SNX-11	Ziconotide	Tx of neuropathic pain and chronic pain, also Tx of spasticity due to spinal cord trauma, and prevention & Tx of brain ischemia caused by CABG
Sodium Bicarbonate	Sodium Bicarbonate	Antacid, Urinary Alkalinizer
Sodium Bicarbonate Injection	Sodium Bicarbonate Inj	Tx of severe acidosis
Sodium Edecrin	Ethacynate Sodium	Diuretic
Sodium Thiosulfate	Sodium Thiosulfate	Antidote

Solagé	Mequinol (4-Hydroxyanisole) & Tretinoin	Solar letigines
Solaraze, (Solarase?)	Diclofenac Sodium Topical	Topical NSAID, Tx of actinic keratoses
Solganal	Aurothioglucose	Antiarthritic
Soltara	Norastemizole	Antihistamine
Solu-Cortef, A-Hydrocort	Hydrocortisone Sodium Succinate	Glucocorticoid
Solu-Medrol, A-MethaPred	Methylprednisolone Sodium Succinate	Glucocorticoid
Soma	Carisoprodol	Skeletal Muscle Relaxant
Soma Compound	Carisoprodol & Aspirin	Muscle Relaxant, Analgesic
Somagard	Deslorelin	Tx of central precocious puberty
SomatoKine	Growth factor/BP3 complex	Tx of osteoporosis
Sonata	Zaleplon	Hypnotic
Sorbitol	Sorbitol	Laxative
Sorbsan, Kaltostat, Kaltostat Fortex	Calcium Alginate Fiber	Protective Dressing
Soriatane	Acitretin	Antipsoriatic,
Sotradecol	Sodium Tetradecyl Sulfate	Sclerosing Agent
Spanidin	Gusperimus	Antirejection
Sparine	Promazine HCl	Antipsychotic Agent
Spectazole	Econazole	Antifungal

Spectracef	Cefditoren pivoxil	Antibiotic
Spectrobid	Bacampicillin HCl	Antibiotic
Spexil	Trospectomycin	Antibiotic
Spiriva	Tiotropium Bromide	Tx of COPD
Sporanox	Itraconazole	Antifungal
SPS, Kayexalate	Sodium Polystyrene Sulfonate	Potassium sequestrant
Stadol	Butorphanol Tartrate	Analgesic, Opiate Partial Agonist
Stadol-NS	Butorphanol Nasal Spray	Analgesic, Opiate Partial Agonist
Staphcillin	Methicillin Sodium	Antibiotic
Staphvax	Staphylococcal Glycoconjugate Vaccine, Bivalent	Vaccine
Star GLA, Ultra GLA, Evening Primrose Oil	Gamma Linolenic Acid	Arthritis, ARDS, PMS, diabetic neuropathy, pruritis, breast cancer, atopic dermatitis, migraine prophylaxis
Starlix	Nateglinide	Antidiabetic
Stedicor	Azimilide	Class III Antiarrhythmic
Stelazine	Trifluoperazine	Antipsychotic, Tranquilizer
Stemgen	Ancestim	Hematopoietic Growth Factor

Steritalc, Sclerosol	Talc, sterile	Malignant pleural effusion
Stilbestrol	Diethylstilbestrol	Estrogen
Stilnox	Stilnox	Short term Tx of sleep disorders
Stilphostrol	Diethylstilbestrol and Diphosphate	Antineoplastic
Stn-KLH	Theratope	Antineoplastic
Streptase, Kabikinase	Streptokinase	Thrombolytic
Streptomycin	Streptomycin Sulfate	Aminoglycoside Antibiotic
Stromectol	Ivermectin	Anthelminic
Sublimaze, Fentanyl Oralet, Actig	Fentanyl Citrate	Narcotic Analgesic
Suboxone	Buprenorphine and Naloxone	Tx of opiate addition
Sucraid	Sacrosidase	Tx of sucrase deficiency (of CSID
Sudafed, Novafed, Genaphed, Halofed, Pseudo-Gest, Sudex, Seudotabs, DeFed-60, Allermed, Sinustop Pro, Novafed, Mini Thin Pseudo, Decofed, Dynafed-60, Cenafed,	Pseudoephedrine HCl (d-Isoephedrine HCl)	Decongestant, Anorectic

Efidac/24, Pseudo		
Sufadiazine	Sufadiazine	Antibiotic, Sulfonamide
Sufenta	Sufentanil Citrate	Narcotic
Sular	Nisoldipine	Antihypertensive, Calcium Channel Blocker
Sulfacet-R, Plexion, Novacet	Sulfacetamide & Sulfur Skin Cleanser	Tx of acne rosacea
Sulfamylon	Mafenide Acetate	Topical Antibacterial
Sulfamylon Solution	Mafenide Solution	Topilal Antiinfective
Summit Extra Strength Caplets	APAP,Aspirin and Caffeine	Analgesic
Sumycin, Achromycin, Tetralan, Panmycin, Robitet, Tetracyn, Teline	Tetracycline	Antibiotic
Supac,	APAP, Aspirin, Caffeine and Calcium Gluconate	Analgesic

Supprelin	Histrelin Acetate	Gonadotropin releasing hormone (GnRH) analog
Suprane	Desflurane	Inhalant Anesthetic
Suprax	Cefixime	Antibiotic
Surfak	Docusate Calcium	Stool Softener
Surfaxin	Lucinactant	For RDS
Surmontil	Trimipramine Mleate	Antidepressant
Surpass	Calcium Carbonate Gum	Antacid
Survanta	Beractant	Lung Surfactant
Sustiva	Efavirenz	Antiviral
Symbicort	Budesonide and Formoterol	Tx of Asthma and COPD
Symlin	Pramlintide Acetate	Tx of diabetes
Symmetrel, Endantadine, 1-adamantanamine	Amantadine HCl	Antiviral, Antiparkinson, treatment of drug-induced extrapyramidal symptoms
Synagis	Palivizumab	Prevention of RSV Infections in premature infants
Synalar, Synemol, Fluoderm, Fluonide	Fluocinolone Acetonide	Anti-inflammitory
Synalgos-DC	Aspirin, Caffeine and Dihydrocodeine	Analgesic combination

Synapton	Physostigmine	Cholinesterase Inhibitor
Synarel	Nafarelin Acetat	Gonadotropin releasing hormone (GnRH) analog
Synercid	Quinupristin and Dalfopristin Injection (Streptogramin class)	Antibiotic
Synthroid, Unithroid, Levothroid, Levoxyl, Thyrox, Levo-T, Eltroxin, Levoxine, Levotec	Levothyroxine Sodium, (T4, L-thyronine)	Thyroid replacement
Syprine, Cuprid	Trientine	Chelating agent
Tace	Chlorotrianisene	Estrogen, Antineoplastic
Tagamet	Cimetidine	H2 Blocker, Anti-ulcer Drug
Talacen	Pentazocine & Acetaminophen	Analgesic Combination
Talwin	Pentazocine	Narcotic Agonist-Antagonist Analgesic
Talwin Compound	Pentazocine and Aspirin	Analgesic Combination
Talwin-NX	Pentazocine and Naloxone	Analgesic
Tambocor	Flecainide Acetate	Group I-C Antiarrhythmic

		Antiviral (Influenza A and B)
Tamiflu	Oseltamivir Phosphate	(Neuraminidase Inhibitor)
Tantum	Benzydamine HCl	Tx of mucositis
TAO	Troleandomycin	Antiinfective
Tapazole	Methimazole	Tx of hyperthyroidism
Taractan	Chlorprothixene	Antipsychotic
Targocid	Teicoplanin	Glycopeptide Antibiotic
Targretin	Bexarotene (LGD1069)	Antineoplastic
Tarka	Trandolapril & Verapamil	Antihypertensive
Tasmar	Tolcapone	Antiparkinson Agent-Catechol O-Methyltransferase (COMT) Inhibitor
Tavist, Antihist-1	Clemastine Fumarate	Antihistamine
Tavist-D	Clemastine and Phenylpropanolamine	Antihistamine, Decongestant
Taxol, Paxene	Paclitaxel	Antineoplastic
Taxol/Herceptin	Paclitaxel and Trastuzumab	Antineoplastic
Taxotere	Docetaxel	Antineoplastic
Tazorac	Tazarotene	Anti-acne, anti-psoriasis
Tebrazid, Zinamide,	Pyrazinamide	Antituberculocis

Pyrazinamide		
Teen, Midol Caplets, Midol RegularStrength Multi-Symptom Caplet	APAP and Pyrilamine	Analgesic
Tegison	Etretinate	Antipsoriasis Agent
Tegretol, Atretol, Epitol, Depito, Carbatrol (ER Caps), Mazepine, Tegretol XR	Carbamazepine	Anticonvulsant
Tegrin	Coal Tar	Dermatologic Agent
Telepaque	Iopanoic Acid	Diagnostic Aid
Temodar, Temodal	Temozolomide	Antineoplastic for astrocytoma & brain carcinoma
Temovate, Clobevate, Dermovate	Clobetasol Propionate	Topical Anti-inflammitory, Corticosteroid
Tempium	Tempium	Smoking cessation
Tenex	Guanfacine HCl	Antihypertensive
Tenoretic	Atenolol & Chlorthalidone	Antihypertensive, Diuretic
Tenormin	Atenolol	ß-Adrenergic Blocker, Antihypertensive
Tenovil	Interleukin-10	Tx of Crohn's Disease Tx of rheumatoid arthritis
Tenovil	rHUIL-10	Tx of rheumatoid

		arthritis
Tenuate, Tepanil, Tenuate Dospan	Diethylpropion HCl	Anorexiant
Tequin	Gatifloxacin	3rd Gen Quinolone Antibiotic
Terazol-7, Terazol-3	Terconazole	Antifungal
Terramycin, Uri-Tet	Oxytetracycline HCl	Antibiotic
Teslac	Testolactone	Antineoplastic, Androgen
Tessalon	Benzonatate	Antitussive
Testandro, Histerone, Tesamone	Testosterone Aq. Susp.	Androgen, short acting
Testopel	Testosterone Pellets	Androgen
Testosterone Propionate	Testosterone Propionate injection (in Oil)	Androgen, short acting
Tet.Tox.	Tetanus Toxoid	Toxoid, Immunization
Teventen/HCTZ	Eprosartan and Hydrochlorothiazide	Antihypertensive
Teveten	Eprosartan	Antihypertensive
Thalomid, Synovir, (Celgene)	Thalidomide	TNF Modifiers, DAARD, Dermatological Agent
Therafectin	Amiprilose	Antiinflammatory
Theraflu	Acetaminophen, pseudoephredrine, dextromethorphan	Analgesic, decongestant, antitussive

Theragyn (HMFG-1)	Yttrium-90-labeled monoclonal antibody	Tx of ovarian and gastric cancer
Thiamine	Vitamin B1	Vitamin
Thioguanine, 6-TG	Thioguanine	Antineoplastic
Thiola	Tiopronin	Cystine-Depleting Agent for prevention of kidney stones
Thioplex	Thiotepa	Antineoplastic
Thiosulfil Forte	Sulfamethizole	Antibacterial
Thorazine, Chlorpromanyl	Chlorpromazine	Antipsychotic, Antiemetic
Threostat	L-Threonine	Tx of ALS and spastic paraparesis
Thrombostat, Thrombinar	Thrombin	Hemostatic
Thypinone, Relefact TRH	Protirelin	Diagnostic Aid
Thyro-Block, Lugol's Solution, Strong Iodine Solution	Potassium Iodide	Thyroid blocking
Thyrogen	Thyrotropin Alfa	Adjunct in the diagnosis of thyroid cancer
Thyroid USP, Armour Thyroid, Thyroid Strong, Thyrar, S-P-T	Thyroid Desiccated	Thyroid Agent
Thytropar, Thyrogen	Thyrotropin	Thyroid Agent
Ticar	Ticarcillin	Antibiotic

Tice BCG, Bacillus of Calmette & Guerin, TheraCys	BCG Vaccine	Vaccine
Ticlid	Ticlopidine	Platelet Aggregation Inhibitor
Tifacogin	Recombinant Tissue Factor Pathway Inhibitor (rTFPI/SC)	Tx of sepsis
Tigan	Trimethobenzamide	Antiemetic
Tikosyn	Dofetilide	Antiarrhythmic
Tilade	Nedocromil Sodium Inh.	Preventive Management of Asthma
Timentin	Ticarcillin & Clavulanic Acid	Antibiotic
Timolide	Hydrochlorothiazide and Timolol Maleate	Antihypertensive
Timolide 10-25	Timolol & HCTZ	Antihypertensive
Timoptic, Timoptic XE, Betimol	Timolol Ophth. Sol.	Antiglaucoma
Tindal	Acetophenazine Maleate	Antipsychotic
Tirazone	Tirapazamine	Cytoxic agent
Titralac Plus	Calcium Carbonate & Simethicone	Antacid, Calcium Supplement
TNKase	Tenecteplase (TNK-tPA)	Thrombolytic - for use in acute MI

TOBI	Tobramycin for Inhalation	Aminoglycoside Antibiotic
TobraDex	Tobramycin & Dexamethasone	Ophth. Anti-infective
Tobrex	Tobramycjn Ophth.	Ophth. Antibacterial
Tofranil, Tofranil-PM, Impril	Imipramine HCl	Antidepressant
Tofranil-PM	Imipramine Pamoate	Antidepressant
Tolectin	Tolmetin	Antiinflammatory, analgesic
Tolinase	Tolazamide	Antidiabetic
Tomudex	Raltitrexed	Antineoplastic
Tonocard	Tocainide	Antiarrhythmic
Tonopaque, Baricon, HD 200 Plus, Barosperse	Barium Sulfate Powder for Suspension	Diagnostic Aid
Topamax	Topiramate	Anticonvulsant
Topicort, Topicort LP	Desoximetasone	Topical Anti-inflammitory
Topicycline Solution, Achromycin Oint	Tetracycline Topical	Antibiotic
Topiglan	Alprostadil (PGE1 Prostaglandin E1) Topical Gel	Tx of erectile dysfunction
Toprol-XL	Metoprolol Succinate	ß-Adrenergic Blocker, Antihypertensive, Antianginal, Post-MI

Toradol	Ketorolac Tromethamine	Analgesic, Anti-inflammitory
Torecan	Thiethylperazine	Antiemetic, Antinauseant
Tornalate Inhaler	Bitolterol Mesylate	Sympathomimetic Agent
t-PA, Activase	Tissue Plasminogen Activator	Thrombolytic
TPO	Thrombopoietin	Platelet growth factor
TPV	Tipranavir	Antiretroviral Agent
Tracrium	Atracurium Besylate	Skeletal Muscle Relaxant
Trancopal	Chlormezanone	Anxiolytic
Transderm-Scop	Scopolamine	Anticholinergic, Antiemetic
Tranxene, Gen-Xene	Clorazepate Dipotassium	Anxiolytic, Sedative, Hypnotic, Anticonvulsant
Trasylol	Aprotinin	Hemostatic
Travatan	Travoprost	Anti-Glaucoma
Trecator-SC	Ethionamide	Antituberulosis Agent
Trelstar Depot	Triptorelin Pamoate	Tx of prostate cancer
Trental	Pentoxifylline	Hemorheologic Agent
Triacana	Tiratricol	Add to levothyroxine in Tx of certain pts with thyroid cancer
Tricor	Fenofibrate	Lipid Regulating Agent
Tridesilon, DesOwen,	Desonide	Corticosteroid

Desocort		
Tridione	Trimethadione	Anticonvulsant
Trihemic 600 Tablets	Hematinic Concentrate with Intrinsic Factor	Hematinic
Trilafon	Perphenazine	Antipsychotic, Phenotriazine
Trileptal	Oxcarbazepine	Anticonvulsant, For siezures and neuroleptic pain.
Trilisate	Choline/Magnesium Salicylate	Analgesic
Tripedia, Acel-Imune, Infanrix, Certiva	Diphtheria, Tetanus Toxoids and Acellular Pertussis Vaccine Adsorbed (DTaP)	Vaccine
Trisenox	Arsenic Trioxide	Tx of promyelocytic leukemia (APL)
Tritec	Ranitidine Bismuth Citrate	Antiulcer
Trizivir	Abacavir, Lamivudine & Zidovudine	Tx of HIV infection
Trobicin	Spectinomycin	Antibiotic
Tronolane, Prax, Tronothane HCl, PrameGel (w/ 0.5% menthol)	Pramoxine HCl	Topical Anesthetic

Trovan	Trovafloxacin	3rd Gen Quinolone Antibiotic
Trovan I.V.	Alatrofloxacin Mesylate	Antibiotic
Trusopt	Dorzolamide HCl	Antiglaucoma
Tubocurarine (Curare)	Tubocurarine	Skeletal muscle relaxant
Tucks	Witch Hazel Wipes	Tx of hemorroids
Tums, OsCal-500, Titralac, Titralac Extra Strength, Caltrate 600, FemCal, Oyst-Cal, Oystercal 500, Cal-Plus, Gencalc 600, Nephro-Calci, Caltrate Jr., Oysco 500, Calci-Chew, Cal-Guard Softgels, Cal Carb-HD, Calci-Mix	Calcium Carbonate	Antacid, Calcium Supplement, Tx of Hyperphosphatemia in Endstage Renal Disease
Tussend	Hydrocodone Pseudoephedrine and Guaifenesin	Antitussive, Decongestant and expectorant
Tussi-12	Carbetapentane, Chlorpheniramine and Phenylephrine	Decongestant, Antitussive and Antihistamine combination
Tussionex	Hydrocodone and Phenyltoloxamine	Antitussive
Tussi-Organidin-S NR, Tussi-	Guaifenesin and Codeine Liquid	Antitussive, Expectorant

Organidin NR Liquid		
Tuss-Ornade, Tussogest	Caraminphen Edisylate and Phenylpropanolamine	Antitussive decongestant
Twinrix	Hepatitis A and B Vaccine	Vaccine
Tylenol Arthritis	Acetaminophen Extended Release	Analgesic/Antipyretic
Tylenol Menstrual Relief	Acetaminophen & Pamabrom	Analgesic & diuretic combination
Tylenol with Codeine	Acetaminophen with Codeine	Analgesic, Narcotic
Tylenol with Codeine Oral Solution, Capital and Codeine Oral Suspension	Acetaminophen with Codeine Oral Liquid	Analgesic, Narcotic
Tylenol, APAP, Atasol, Panadol, Tempra	Acetaminophen	Analgesic/Antipyretic
Tylenol-PM	Acetaminophen and diphenhydramine	Combination analgesic and sleep aid (sedating antihistamine)
Tyzine, Visine	Tetrahydrozoline	Ophthalmic Vasoconstrictor
UbiQGel, Q-Gel Forte, Coenzyme Q-10, CoQ10	Ubiquinone	Mitochondrial cytopathies

Ucephan, Ammonul	Sodium Benzoate & Sodium Phenylacetate	Tx of hyperammonemia
UFT	Tegafur	Antineoplastic for metastatic colorectal cancer
UFT (4:1 molar ratio)	Tegafur and uracil	Antineoplastic for metastatic colorectal cancer
Ultiva	Remifentanil HCl	Analgesic, I.V. Anesthetic
Ultracaine	Articaine	Local anesthetic
Ultracet	Tramadol and Acetaminophen	Analgesic, Short term (5 days or less) mgmt of acute pain
Ultram	Tramadol	Analgesic
Ultram-SR	Tramadol Extended Release	Analgesic
Ultravate	Halobetasol Propionate	Antiinflammatory
Unasyn	Ampicillin Sodium & Sulbactam Sodium	Antibiotic
Uni-Cap, Theragran, Hexavitamin	Multi-Vitamin	Vitamin
Unicap-T, Theragran-M	Multi-Vitamin with Minerals	Vitamin
Unicard	Dilevalol	Noncardioselective ß-adrenergic blocker
Uniretic	Moexipril & HCTZ	Antihypertensive

Unisom, Decapryn, Sleep Aid	Doxylamine Succinte	Sedative
Univasc	Moexipril	Antihypertensive
Uprima, Purim	Apomorphine HCl	For Erectile Dysfunction, Tx of Parkinson's Disease
Ureaphil	Urea Injection	Osmotic Diuretic
Urecholine, Duvoid, Motonachoh	Bethanechol Chloride	Parasympathomimetic Agent
Uricase, Uricozyme	Urate Oxidase	Reduction of uric acid levels associated with chemotherapy (Uricolytic)
Urised	Methylene Blue, Atropine, Methenamine, Phenyl Salicylate, Benzoic acid and Hyoscyamine	Urinary Antiinfective
Urispas	Flavoxate HCl	Smooth Muscle Relaxant, Urinary Antispasmotic
Urobiotic-250	Oxytetracycline, Sulfamethizole & Phenazopyridine	Urinary Antiinfective, Analgesic
Urocit-K	Potassium Citrate	Urinary Alkalinizer
Urolene Blue, Methblue	Methylene Blue	Cyanide Antidote (Methmoglobinemia), GU Antiseptic
Uticort	Betamethasone	Antiinflammatory

	Benzoate	
Vagifem	Estradiol Hemihydrate	Hormone
Vagistat-1, Gynecure, Monistat-1	Tioconazole	Antifungal
Valcyte, Cymeval	Valganciclovir	Antiviral
Valertest, Androgyn LA, Deladumone	Estradiol Cypionate and Testosterone Enanthate	Estrogen & Androgen Combination
Valisone, Betarex, Celestone	Betamethasone Valerate	Topical Anti-Inflammatory
Valium, Diastat, Vivol	Diazepam	Anxiolytic, Skeletal Muscle Relaxant, Anticonvulsant
Valmid	Ethinamate	Hypnotic, Sedative
Valstar	Valrubicin	Tx of refractory bladder cancer
Valtrex	Valacyclovir	Antiviral
Vancocin, Vancoled, Lyphocin	Vancomycin	Antibiotic (Glycopeptide Class)
Vaniqa	Eflornithine HCl Topical	Hair Growth Blocker
Vanlev	Omapatrilat	Antihypertensive & Tx of CHF
Vanquish Caplets	APAP, Aspirin, Caffeine and Magnesium Hydroxide	Analgesic
Vansil	Oxamniquine	Anthelminic

Vantin, Banan	Cefpodoxime Proxetil	Antibiotic
Varivax	Varicella Vaccine	Vaccine
Vascor	Bepridil	Calcium Channel Blocker, Antiangina
Vascoray	Iothalmate Meglumine 52% and Iothalamate Sodium 26%	Diagnostic Aid
Vaseretic	Enalapril Maleate & Hydrochlorothiazide	Antihypertensive
Vasocidin, Cetapred, Isopto Cetapred, Sulfapred, Blephamide	Sulfacetamide & Prednisolone	Ophth. Antibacterial, Antiinflammatory
Vasocon-A	Naphazoline and Antazoline	Ophth. Vasoconstrictor
Vasodilan, Voxsuprine	Isoxsuprine HCl	Peripheral Vasodilator
Vasomax	Phentolamine Mesylate Oral	Tx of male erectile dysfunction
Vasosulf	Sulfacetamide and Phenylepherine	Sulfonamide and decongestant
Vasotec	Enalapril Maleate	Antihypertensive, Heart Failure Drug
Vasotec I.V.	Enalaprilat	Antihypertensive
Vasoxyl	Methoxamine HCl	Vasopressor
VCF	Nonoxynol 9	Spermicide

	Vaginal Film	Contraceptive
V-Echinocandin	Anidulafungin	Antifungal
Velban, VLB	Vinblastine Sulfate	Antineoplastic
Veletri	Tezosentan	Tx of acute heart failure
Veloda	Interferon Alfa	Tx of Sjogren's Syndrome
Velosef	Cephradine	Antibiotic
Velosulin BR	Insulin Regular, Human Buffered (rDNA origin)	Hormone, diabetes mellitus
Venofer, (Iron Sucrose Injection, Iron Saccharate, Iron III Hydroxide Sucrose Complex)	Ferric Hydroxide Sucrose Complex	Hematinic, For iron deficiency in patients undergoing chronic hemodialysis and receiving erythropoietin.
VePesid, VP-16, Toposak	Etoposide	Antineoplastic
Vermox	Mebendazole	Anthelminic
Versed	Midazolam HCl	Sedative (for conscious sedation)
Vesprin	Triflupromazine HCl	Antiemetic, Antipsychotic
Vexol	Rimexolone	Corticosteroid
Vfend	Voriconazole	Antifungal
Viagra	Silenafil Citrate	For Erectile Dysfunction
Viagra Zydis	Silenafil Citrate, Rapid Disolving	Phosphodiesterase-5 Inhibitor For Erectile Dysfunction

Vianain	Ananain, comosain	Enzymatic debridement of severe burns
Vibramycin	Doxycycline Calcium	Antibiotic
Vibramycin, Monodox, Adoxa	Doxycycline Monohydrate	Antibiotic
Vibramycin, Periostat, Doxychel, Doxy, Doryx, Monodox	Doxycycline Hyclate	Antibiotic
Vicks Inhaler	l-desoxyephedrine	Decongestant
Vicodin, Lortab, Hy-Phen, Anexia, Co-Gesic, Hy-Phen, Norco, Lorcet	Hydrocodone and Acetaminophen	Analgesic, Narcotic
Vicodin, Lortab, Lorcet, Anexsia, Bancap HC, Ceta-Plus, Co-Gesic, Dolacet, Dolagesic, Dolorex Forte, Duocet, Allay, Zydone, Hydrocet, Hydrogesic, Hy-Phen, Lorcet-HD, Lorcet Plus, Lortab Elixir, Margesic-H, Norco, Panacet, Polygesic, Stagesic, Vanacet,	Acetaminophen with Hydrocodone	Analgesic, Narcotic, HB/APAP

T-Gesic, Ugesic, Vidone, Vicodin ES, Vicodin HP		
Vicoprofen	Hydrocodone and Ibuprofen	Narcotic Analgesic
Videx, Videx QD, Videx EC, ddI	Didanosine	Antiviral
VIL	Valine, isoleucine and leucine	Hyperphenylalaninemia
Vioform, Iodochlorhydroxyquin	Clioquinol	Topical Antiinfective
Vioxx	Rofecoxib	Anti-inflammatory, analgesic, NSAID (COX-2 Inhibitor)
Viozan	AR-C68397	Tx of COPD
Viprinex	Ancrod	Anticoagulation in heparin-intolerant patients undergoing cardiopulmonary

		bypass
Vira-A	Vidarabine (Adenine Arabinoside, Ara-A)	EENT Antiviral
Viracept	Nelfinavir Mesylate	Antiviral
Viramune	Nevirapine	Antiviral
Virazole	Ribavirin	Antiviral
Viroptic	Trifluridine (Trifluorothymidine)	EENT Antiviral
Visken	Pindolol	ß-Adrenergic Blocker, Antihypertensive
Vistaril Oral	Hydroxyzine Pamoate	Sedative, Antipruritic, Antianxiety Agent
Vistide, Forvade	Cidofovir	Antiviral
Visudyne	Verteporfin	Tx of age-related macular degeneration
Vitamin A	Vitamin A	
Vitamin B-12, Nascobal	Cyanocobalamin	Vitamin
Vitamin C	Ascorbic Acid	Vitamin
Vitamin-E	Alpha Tocopherol	Vitamin
Vitron-C	Ferrous Fumarate with Vitamin C	Hematinic
Vivactil	Protriptyline HCl	Antidepressant
Voltaren	Diclofenac Sodium	Antiinflammatory

Voltaren, Vofenal	Diclofenac	Ophthalmic NSAID
Vontrol	Diphenidol	Antiemetic, Meniere's Syndrome, Antivertigo
VoSol-HC Otic	Acetic Acid & Hydrocortisone	Otic Antiinfective, Antiinflammatory
Vumon Injection	Teniposide	Acute lymphocytic leukemia
VZIG	Varicella-Zoster Immune Globulin	Immunoglobulin
Welchol	Colesevelam HCl	Bile Acid Sequestrant
Welcovorin	Leucovorin Calcium, Folinic Acid, Citrovorum Factor	Leucovorin 'rescue' after high-dose methotrexate therapy
Wellbutrin, Zyban	Bupropion	Antidepressant, Smoking sessation agent (Zyban)
Wellferon Injection	Interferon Alfa-n1 (lymphoblastoid)	Treatment of chronic hepatitis C
Westcort, Dermatop	Hydrocortisone Valerate	Topical Antiinflammatory
Wigraine, Ercaf, Gotamine, Cafergot	Ergotamine Tartrate & Caffeine Tablets	Antimigraine
WinRho SDF, RhoGAM, BayRho-D, MICRhoGAM	Rho(D) Immune Ghobulin Intravenous (Human)	Biologic response modifier
Winstrol	Stanozolol	Anabolic Steroid
Wyamine Sulfate	Mephentermine Sulfate	Vasopressor

Wydase	Hyaluronidase	Absorption Facilitator
Wygesic	Propoxyphene HCl and Acetaminophen	Analgesic, Opioid Agonist
Wytensin	Guanabenz Acetate	Antihypertensive
Xalatan	Latanoprost	Antiglaucoma
Xalcom	Latanoprost and Timolol Ophthalmic Sol	Antiglaucoma
Xanax, Alprazolam Intensol	Alprazolam	Anxiolytic
Xanelim	Efalizumab	Tx of psoriasis
Xanomeline	Xanomeline	M1 muscarinic receptor agonist for Tx of Alzheimer's
Xatral OD	Alfuzosin	Tx of BPH
Xeloda	Capecitabine	Antineoplastic, Tx of colon cancer
Xenical	Orlistat (tetrahydrolipstatin)	Weight Loss Agent
Xeroform	Bismuth Tribromophenate	Protective Dressing
Xilep	Rufinamide	Antiepileptic
Xolair	Omalizumab (rhuMAb-E25)	Tx of asthma
Xopenex	Levalbuterol	Bronchodilator
Xubix	Sibrafiban	Investigational for Angina, PCI, and MI
Xylocaine	Lidocaine Intravenous	Group I-B Antiarrhythmic

Xylocaine, Numby Stuff, Nervocaine	Lidocaine HCl	Local Anesthetic
Xyrem	Sodium Oxybate and Sodium Gamma Hydroxybutyrate	Tx of narcolepsy, alcohol withdrawal
Xyvion	Tibolone (OD-14)	Synthetic steroid analog
Yasmin 28	Drospirenone and Ethinyl Estradiol	Oral Contraseptive
YF-Vax	Yellow Fever Vaccine	Vaccine
Yodoxin, Diodoquin, diiodohydroxyquin	Iodoquinol	Amebicide
Yutopar	Ritodrine HCl	Uterine Relaxant
Zadaxin	Thymalfasin	Antineoplastic, Antiviral
Zaditor	Ketotifen fumarate	Ophth. Antihistamine
Zagam	Sparfloxacin	Quinolone Antibiotic
Zanaflex	Tizanidine	Skeletal muscle relaxant
Zanosar	Streptozocin	Antineoplastic
Zantac, Zantac-75	Ranitidine	Antiulcer
Zarontin	Ethosuximide	Anticonvulsant
Zaroxolyn, Mykrox	Metolazone	Diuretic
Zebeta	Bisoprolol Fumarate	ß-Adrenergic Blocker, Antihypertensive
Zefazone	Cefmetazole	Antibiotic

Zelapar	Selegiline Rapid Dissolving Tab	Tx of Parkinson's Disease
Zelmac	Tegaserod	For irritable bowel syndrome also Tx of GERD & Dyspepsia
Zemplar	Paricalcitol	Vitamin D analog
Zemuron	Rocuronium	Neuromuscular Blocking Agent
Zenapax, Humanized anti-tac	Daclizumab	Immunosuppressive
Zendra	Clomethiazole	Tx of acute ischemic stroke
Zerit	Stavudine (d4T)	Antiviral
Zerit ER, d4T	Stavudine extended release	Antiviral
Zevalin (IDEC-Y2B8)	Ibritumomab	Antineoplastic, Tx of non-Hodgkins Lymphoma (NHL)
Zevelin	Ibritumomab Tiuxetan	Tx of refractory non-Hodgkin's
Ziac	Bisoprolol Fumarate & Hydrochlorothiazide	Antihypertensive
Ziagen	Abacavir	Antiviral
Zinc Sulfate	Zinc Sulfate	Dietary supplement
Zinecard	Dexrazoxane	Cytoprotective Agent
Ziracin	Everninomicin	Antibiotic
Zithromax	Azithromycin	Antibiotic

Zixoryn	Flumecinol	Tx of newborn hyperbilirubinemia unresponsive to phototherapy
Zocor	Simvastatin	Antihyperlipidemic
Zofran, Zofran ODT	Ondansetron HCl	Antiemetic
Zoladex	Goserelin	Antineoplastic
Zoloft	Sertraline HCl	Antidepressant, Tx of panic disorder or PTSD
Zomaril	Iloperidone	Tx of schizophrenia
Zometa	Zoledronic Acid	Tx of tumor-induced hypercalcemia
Zomig, Zomig-ZMT	Zolmitriptan	Antimigraine
Zonalon, Prudoxin	Doxepin HCl Topical	Antihistamine
Zonegran, Exegran	Zonisamide (Valphenytoin)	Antiepleptic, Sulfonamide Class
Zostrix, Zostrix-HP	Capsaicin Cream	Topical Analgesic
Zosyn, Tazocin	Piperacillin Sodium & Tazobactam Sodium	Antibiotic
Zovant, (rhAPC)	Drotrecogin Alfa (Activated Protein C, Recombinant Human)	Tx of severe sepsis

Zovant, rhAPC	Recombinant Human Activated Protein C (Drotrecogin alpha)	Tx of severe sepsis
Zovirax, Avirax	Acyclovir (Acycloguanosine)	Antiviral
Zyflo	Zileuton	Antiasthmatic
Zyloprim Injection, Aloprim	Allopurinol Sodium	Uricostatic
Zyloprim, Purinol, Alloprim	Allopurinol	Antigout Agent (Uricostatic)
Zyprexa, Zyprexa Zydis	Olanzapine	Antipsychotic Agent
Zyrkamine	Mitoguazone	Tx of non-Hodgkin's lymphoma
Zyrtec D	Cetirizine and	Antihistamine and decongestant combination
Zyrtec, Reactine	Cetirizine	Antihistamine
Zyvox	Linezolid	Antibiotic

One Final Thought

There will be days where you will feel that you are being blamed for everything wrong with the world. There will be days where you are rehearsing for a less stressful job,
"do you want fries with that"
And there will be days that you go home with a smile on your face that no one understands. That smile is the satisfaction of knowing you and your actions kept somebody alive, eased someone's pain, made someone's life a little better, or even helped someone go to heaven peacefully. Live for those days and never let anyone take your smile away.

God bless you – you are a nurse